Fit Feast

Your Guide to 40 Low-Calorie, High-Nutrition Main Courses

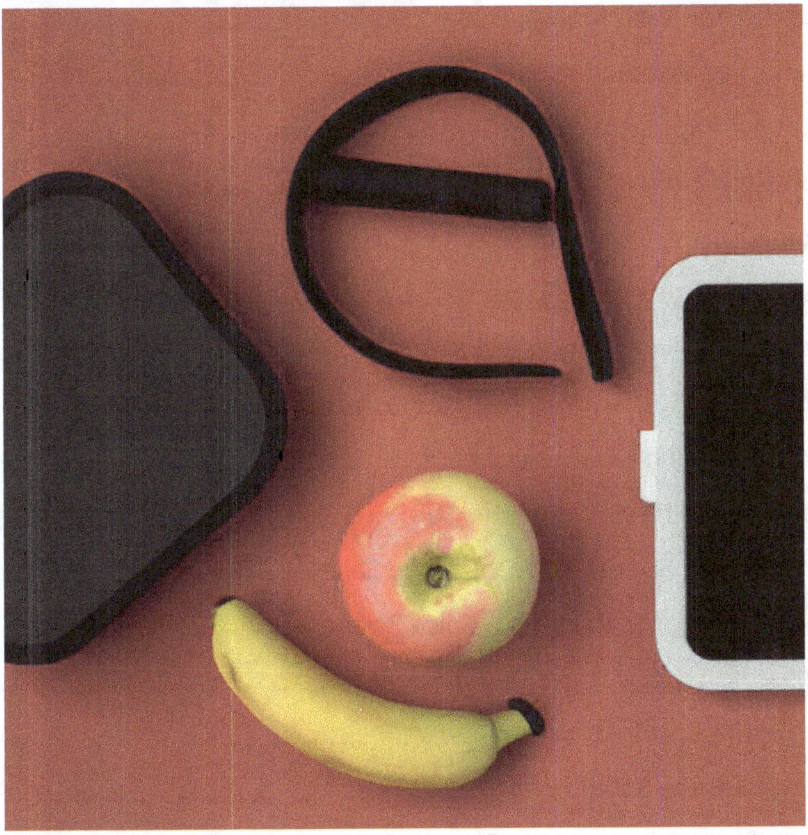

Wellington Barreto

Table of Contents

Introduction

Welcome to "Fit Feast," your ultimate companion on a nourishing voyage towards wellness, health, and of course, deliciousness. This book is a careful curation of 40 exquisite, low-calorie, high-nutrition main course recipes crafted with attention to the needs of fitness enthusiasts, health warriors, and anyone seeking a vibrant, balanced lifestyle. If you're yearning to add a dash of wholesome yet mouth-watering variety to your meals while keeping a keen eye on your caloric intake, you have arrived at your destination.

"Fit Feast" is born out of a profound belief that wholesome nutrition and mouth-watering meals should be more than just occasional treats. We deserve to indulge in them every day, without compromising our fitness goals or feeling guilty about those extra calories. Each recipe in this collection is lovingly designed to balance low calorie count with high nutritional value, fulfilling taste, and ample satisfaction.

This recipe book moves beyond the conventional perception of low-calorie meals as bland salads or tasteless, portion-controlled dishes. It offers you a palette of flavours from all around the world, each recipe boasting its unique profile yet unifying in their commitment to your health. The recipes are not only about staying within your calorie count but are also about providing you with a powerful punch of essential nutrients. Every dish you create from this book is a step towards enhancing your health, boosting your energy, and maintaining a radiant glow from within.

"Fit Feast" explores the breadth and depth of dietary options, catering to various tastes, preferences, and dietary requirements. We have included vegetarian, vegan, dairy-free, and meat-based meals to ensure no one feels left out. This approach is to empower you with choices and let you take control of your diet while enjoying a diverse range of foods.

One key attribute of this book is its simplicity. Each of our 40 recipes is meticulously detailed, easy to follow, and requires ingredients that are accessible in most local markets. No professional culinary skills are required—just a sprinkle of passion, a dollop of commitment, and a hunger for healthy, satisfying food. We've also added prep and cooking times to help you plan your meals seamlessly.

Moreover, alongside each recipe, you'll find the caloric and nutritional breakdown of the meal. This will empower you with the knowledge of exactly what you are consuming, which is a crucial aspect of maintaining a healthy lifestyle. You'll also find handy tips and tricks, serving suggestions, and variations to help you tailor each dish to your unique preferences and dietary needs.

Food is more than fuel; it's an experience, a comfort, a love language. And we firmly believe that embarking on a journey to health and fitness should not require giving up on the joy of eating. This is why "Fit Feast" is so much more than a cookbook; it's a celebration of food, health, and life.

Whether you're a seasoned gym-goer, a yoga lover, a long-distance runner, or someone simply seeking to maintain a healthier lifestyle, "Fit Feast" has a seat for you at the table. This collection of 40 low-calorie, high-nutrition mains is a testament to the fact that healthy eating can be diverse, satisfying, and above all, delectably enjoyable.

So, get ready to embark on this flavourful journey to wellness. As you flip through the pages, you'll find more than just recipes; you'll discover a new perspective on food, health, and fitness. Enjoy the tantalizing tastes, relish in the satisfaction of nourishing your body, and celebrate the joy of achieving your fitness goals without compromising on the delicious journey.

Quinoa Stuffed Bell Peppers

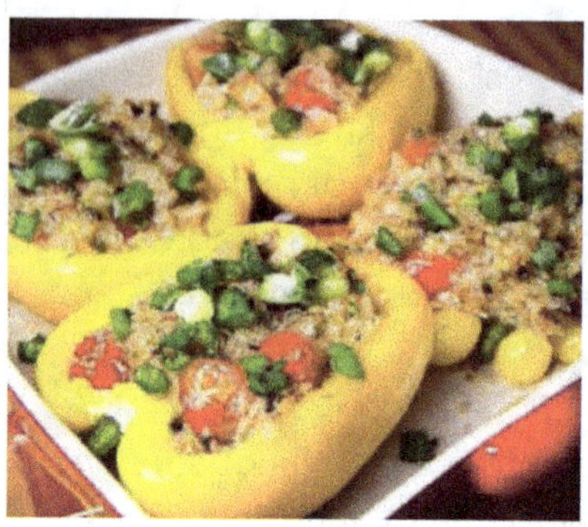

Portion Size: 4 servings

Macronutrient Breakdown (per serving):

- Calories: 350
- Protein: 15g
- Carbohydrates: 45g
- Fat: 12g
- Fibre: 8g

Ingredients:

- 1 cup quinoa (uncooked)
- 2 cups vegetable broth
- 4 large bell peppers (assorted colours)
- 1 small onion, finely chopped
- 1 can (15 oz) black beans, drained and rinsed
- 1 cup corn kernels (fresh or frozen)
- 1 cup cherry tomatoes, halved
- 1/2 cup cilantro, chopped
- 1 teaspoon ground cumin
- 1 teaspoon chili powder
- 1/2 teaspoon garlic powder
- Salt and pepper to taste
- 1 cup shredded cheddar cheese
- 1 tablespoon olive oil

Instructions:

1. Preheat your oven to 375°F (190°C).
2. In a medium saucepan, combine quinoa and vegetable broth, then bring to a boil. Lower the heat, cover, and simmer for 15 minutes, or until the quinoa is cooked and has absorbed the broth.

3. Cut the tops off the bell peppers and remove seeds and membranes. Place the peppers in a baking dish and set aside.
4. In a large bowl, combine cooked quinoa, onion, black beans, corn, cherry tomatoes, cilantro, cumin, chili powder, garlic powder, salt, and pepper.
5. Stuff each bell pepper with the quinoa mixture, filling them evenly.
6. Top each pepper with shredded cheddar cheese and drizzle with olive oil.
7. Cover the baking dish with foil and bake for 25 minutes. Remove the foil and bake for an additional 5-10 minutes, or until the cheese is melted and the peppers are tender.
8. Serve immediately and enjoy!

Greek Yogurt Chicken Salad

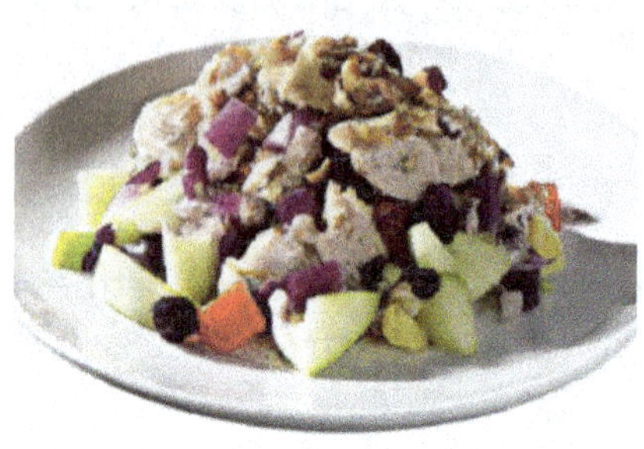

Portion Size: 4 servings

Macronutrient Breakdown (per serving):

- Calories: 265
- Protein: 28g
- Carbohydrates: 15g
- Fat: 10g
- Fibre: 3g

Ingredients:

- 2 cups cooked chicken breast, shredded
- 1/2 cup plain Greek yogurt
- 1/4 cup mayonnaise
- 1 apple, diced
- 1/2 cup red grapes, halved
- 1/4 cup sliced almonds
- 1/4 cup chopped green onions
- 1/4 cup chopped celery
- Salt and pepper to taste

Instructions:

1. In a large mixing bowl, combine Greek yogurt and mayonnaise until smooth.
2. Add in the shredded chicken, apple, grapes, almonds, green onions, and celery. Mix well.
3. Season with salt and pepper to taste.
4. Refrigerate for at least 30 minutes to allow flavours to meld.
5. Serve on whole-grain bread or over a bed of mixed greens.

Turkey & Veggie Stir-Fry

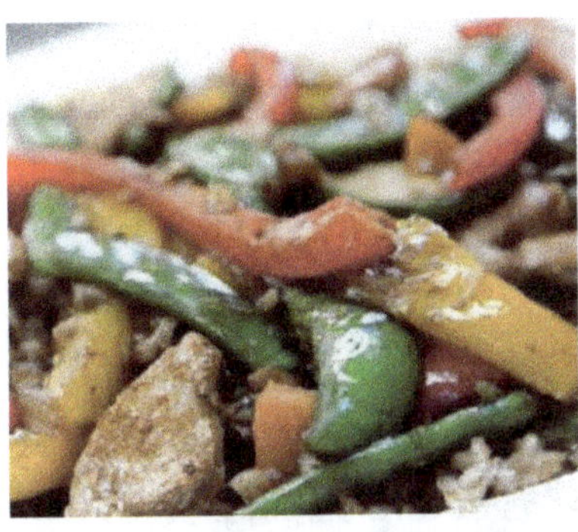

Portion Size: 4 servings

Macronutrient Breakdown (per serving):

- Calories: 330
- Protein: 30g
- Carbohydrates: 25g
- Fat: 12g
- Fibre: 6g

Ingredients:
- 1 pound lean ground turkey
- 1 tablespoon olive oil
- 2 cloves garlic, minced
- 1 small onion, diced
- 1 medium zucchini, sliced into half-moons
- 1 medium red bell pepper, sliced into thin strips
- 1 medium yellow bell pepper, sliced into thin strips
- 1/2 cup snap peas, trimmed
- 1/4 cup low-sodium soy sauce
- 1 tablespoon honey
- 1 teaspoon corn starch
- 1/4 teaspoon ground ginger
- Salt and pepper to taste
- 2 tablespoons green onions, chopped (for garnish)
- 1 tablespoon sesame seeds (for garnish)

Instructions:

1. In a large skillet or wok, heat the olive oil over medium heat. Add the garlic and onion and sauté until fragrant and the onion becomes translucent, about 2-3 minutes.

2. Add the ground turkey to the skillet, breaking it up as it cooks. Cook until the turkey is browned and cooked through, about 5-7 minutes. Drain any excess fat.

3. Add the zucchini, red and yellow bell peppers, and snap peas to the skillet. Cook, stirring occasionally, for 5-7 minutes, or until the vegetables are tender-crisp.

4. In a small bowl, whisk together the soy sauce, honey, corn starch, and ground ginger. Pour the sauce over the turkey and veggie mixture, stirring well to coat.

5. Cook for an additional 2-3 minutes or until the sauce thickens.

6. Season with salt and pepper to taste.

7. Garnish with green onions and sesame seeds before serving. Enjoy with a side of brown rice or quinoa for a complete meal.

Roasted Chickpea & Cauliflower Buddha Bowl

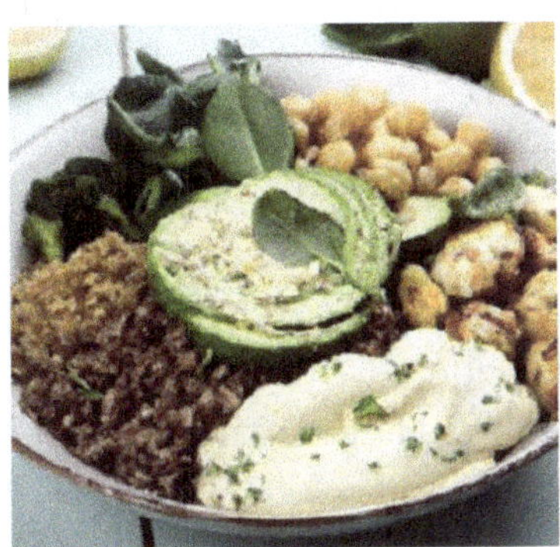

Portion Size: 4 servings

Macronutrient Breakdown (per serving):

- Calories: 400
- Protein: 18g
- Carbohydrates: 55g
- Fat: 14g
- Fibre: 12g

Ingredients:

- 1 can (15 oz) chickpeas, drained, rinsed, and patted dry
- 1 medium head cauliflower, cut into florets
- 1 tablespoon olive oil
- 1/2 teaspoon ground cumin
- 1/2 teaspoon smoked paprika
- Salt and pepper to taste
- 4 cups baby spinach
- 1 cup cooked quinoa
- 1 avocado, sliced
- 1/4 cup hummus
- Lemon wedges for serving

Instructions:

1. Preheat the oven to 425°F (220°C). Line a baking sheet with parchment paper.
2. In a large bowl, toss the chickpeas and cauliflower florets with olive oil, cumin, smoked paprika, salt, and pepper until well coated.
3. Spread the chickpeas and cauliflower evenly on the prepared baking sheet.

4.   Roast in the oven for 25-30 minutes, or until the chickpeas are crispy and the cauliflower is tender and slightly charred. Stir halfway through cooking.
5.   To assemble the Buddha bowls, divide the baby spinach and cooked quinoa among four serving bowls.
6.   Top each bowl with an equal portion of the roasted chickpea and

Note: Feel free to customize your Buddha bowl by adding your favourite roasted or raw vegetables, grains, or protein sources. This versatile dish can be adapted to suit your taste preferences and dietary needs.

Grilled Salmon with Mango Salsa

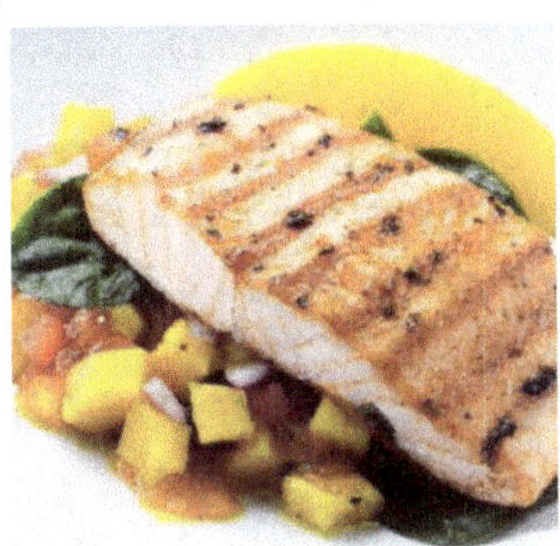

Portion Size: 4 servings

Macronutrient Breakdown (per serving):

- Calories: 370
- Protein: 34g
- Carbohydrates: 25g
- Fat: 15g
- Fibre: 4g

Ingredients:

- 4 salmon fillets (6 oz each)
- Salt and pepper to taste
- 1 tablespoon olive oil
- 1 large ripe mango, diced
- 1 small red bell pepper, diced
- 1/2 small red onion, finely chopped
- 1/4 cup chopped fresh cilantro
- 1 jalapeño, seeds removed and finely chopped (optional)
- Juice of 1 lime
- 1/4 teaspoon ground cumin

Instructions:

1. Preheat your grill to medium-high heat.
2. Season the salmon fillets with salt and pepper and brush with olive oil.
3. In a medium bowl, combine the diced mango, red bell pepper, red onion, cilantro, jalapeño (if using), lime juice, and ground cumin. Mix well and set aside.
4. Grill the salmon fillets for 4-5 minutes per side or until cooked to your desired doneness.
5. Remove the salmon from the grill and let it rest for a couple of minutes.

6.   Top each salmon fillet with a generous scoop of mango salsa.
7.   Serve immediately with a side of steamed vegetables or a mixed
        green salad. Enjoy!

Chicken, Broccoli, and Brown Rice Casserole

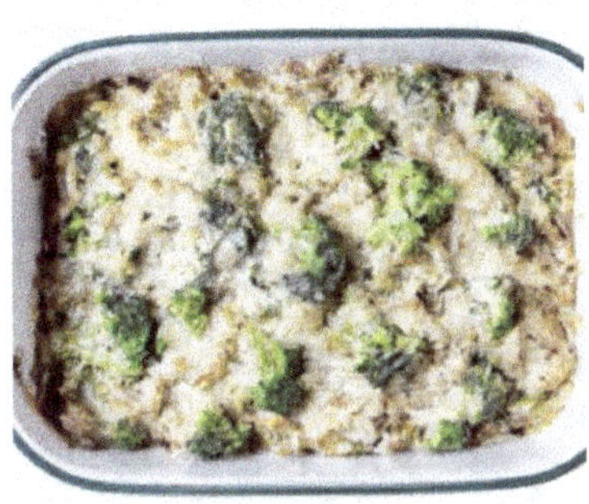

Portion Size: 6 servings

Macronutrient Breakdown (per serving):

- Calories: 410
- Protein: 32g
- Carbohydrates: 45g
- Fat: 12g
- Fibre: 4g

Ingredients:

- 1 cup uncooked brown rice
- 2 cups low-sodium chicken broth
- 2 cups cooked chicken breast, cubed
- 4 cups broccoli florets, steamed
- 1 can (10.5 oz) condensed cream of chicken soup (low sodium)
- 1/2 cup plain Greek yogurt
- 1/2 cup milk (any type)
- 1 teaspoon garlic powder
- 1 teaspoon onion powder
- 1/2 teaspoon dried thyme
- Salt and pepper to taste
- 1 cup shredded cheddar cheese
- 1/4 cup grated Parmesan cheese

Instructions:

1. Preheat your oven to 350°F (175°C).
2. In a medium saucepan, combine the brown rice and chicken broth. Bring to a boil, then reduce the heat, cover, and simmer for 45 minutes, or until the rice is cooked and has absorbed the broth.
3. In a large mixing bowl, combine the cooked chicken, steamed broccoli, cooked brown rice, cream of chicken soup, Greek yogurt,

milk, garlic powder, onion powder, dried thyme, salt, and pepper. Mix well.
4. Pour the mixture into a greased 9x13-inch baking dish.
5. Top with the shredded cheddar cheese and grated Parmesan cheese.
6. Bake for 25-30 minutes or until the cheese is melted and bubbly.
7. Let the casserole rest for 5 minutes before serving. Enjoy!

Beef and Vegetable Stir-Fry

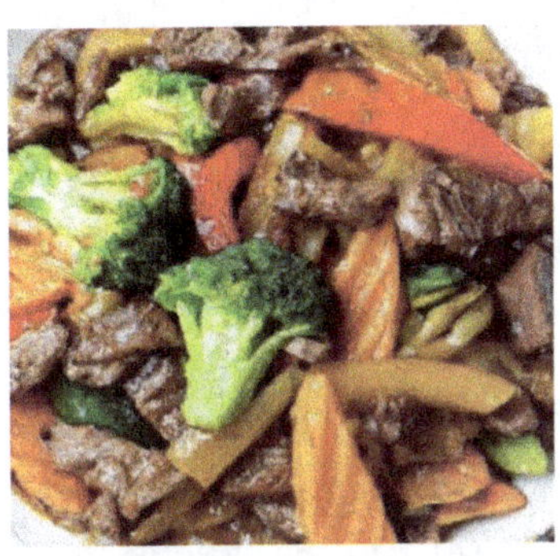

Portion Size: 4 servings

Macronutrient Breakdown (per serving):

- Calories: 420
- Protein: 35g
- Carbohydrates: 40g
- Fat: 14g
- Fibre: 5g

Ingredients:

- 1 pound beef sirloin, thinly sliced into strips
- 2 tablespoons vegetable oil, divided
- 1 medium red bell pepper, sliced into thin strips
- 1 medium yellow bell pepper, sliced into thin strips
- 1 large carrot, julienned
- 2 cups broccoli florets
- 1/4 cup low-sodium

Instructions:

1. First, make sure all your vegetables and beef are cut and ready. Prepping everything before you start cooking will make the process smoother.
2. Heat 1 tablespoon of the vegetable oil in a large skillet or wok over medium-high heat. Add the beef strips and stir fry for about 2-3 minutes or until it's mostly cooked through. Remove the beef from the skillet and set it aside on a separate plate.
3. In the same skillet, add the remaining 1 tablespoon of vegetable oil. Add the sliced bell peppers and julienned carrots. Stir fry these for about 2 minutes.
4. Next, add the broccoli florets to the skillet. If your skillet is becoming dry, you can add a little bit of water to help steam the broccoli.

Continue to stir fry until the vegetables are tender, but still crispy, about 2-3 more minutes.

5.   Return the beef to the skillet with the vegetables. Add the 1/4 cup of low-sodium soy sauce. Stir everything together and continue to cook for another 2 minutes, or until the beef is cooked to your liking and the sauce has heated through.

6.   Optional: Add minced garlic or grated ginger at the same time you add the soy sauce for added flavour. You can also sprinkle sesame seeds on top before serving.

7.   Serve the stir fry hot over rice or noodles if you prefer. Enjoy!

Please make sure to adjust the cooking times based on your stove and how you like your vegetables and beef cooked. Cooking times can vary.

Chicken and Spinach Stuffed Portobello Mushrooms

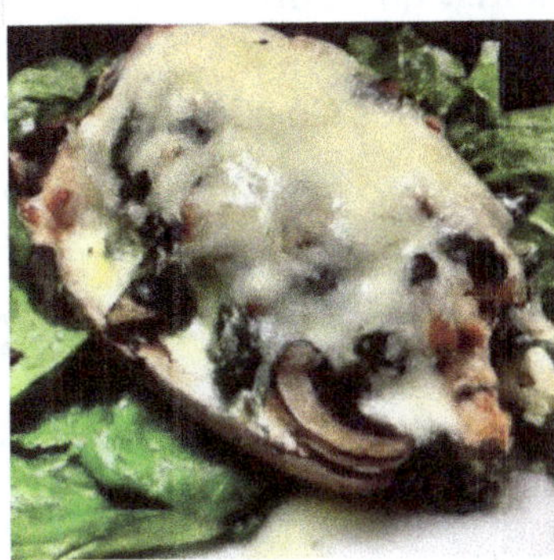

Portion Size: 4 servings

Macronutrient Breakdown (per serving):

- Calories: 310
- Protein: 35g
- Carbohydrates: 11g
- Fat: 14g
- Fibre: 3g

Ingredients:

- 4 large Portobello mushroom caps, cleaned and stems removed
- 1 pound boneless, skinless chicken breast, cooked and diced
- 2 cups fresh spinach, cooked and roughly chopped
- 2 cloves garlic, minced
- 1/2 cup grated Parmesan cheese
- Salt and pepper, to taste
- 1 tablespoon olive oil
- 1 cup shredded mozzarella cheese

Instructions:

1. Preheat your oven to 375°F (190°C). Line a baking sheet with parchment paper or aluminium foil.
2. In a medium bowl, combine the diced chicken, cooked spinach, minced garlic, and Parmesan cheese. Season the mixture with salt and pepper, to taste.
3. Brush the Portobello mushroom caps with olive oil and place them gill-side up on the prepared baking sheet.
4. Spoon the chicken and spinach mixture evenly into each mushroom cap.

5.   Top each stuffed mushroom with an equal amount of shredded mozzarella cheese.

6.   Bake the stuffed mushrooms for 20-25 minutes or until the mushrooms are tender and the cheese is melted and bubbly.

7.   Remove the mushrooms from the oven, let them rest for a few minutes, and serve immediately. Enjoy your delicious Chicken and Spinach Stuffed Portobello Mushrooms!

Lemon Herb Grilled Shrimp and Asparagus

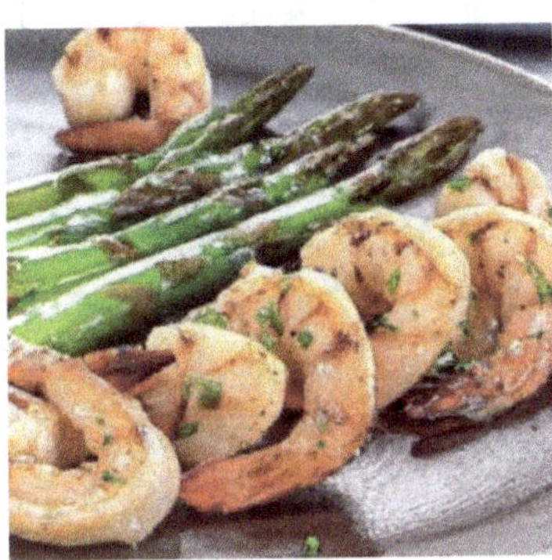

Portion Size: 4 servings

Macronutrient Breakdown (per serving):

- Calories: 260
- Protein: 30g
- Carbohydrates: 8g
- Fat: 11g
- Fibre: 3g

Ingredients:

- 1 pound large shrimp, peeled and deveined
- 1 pound asparagus spears, trimmed
- 3 tablespoons olive oil
- Zest and juice of 1 lemon
- 2 cloves garlic, minced
- 1 tablespoon chopped fresh parsley
- 1 tablespoon chopped fresh basil
- Salt and pepper, to taste
- Wooden or metal skewers (if using wooden skewers, soak them in water for 30 minutes)

Instructions:

1. In a small bowl, whisk together olive oil, lemon zest, lemon juice, minced garlic, parsley, basil, salt, and pepper.
2. Place the shrimp in a shallow dish or a large zip-top plastic bag. Pour half of the marinade over the shrimp, making sure they're well-coated. Refrigerate for 15-30 minutes.
3. In another shallow dish or zip-top plastic bag, place the asparagus spears. Pour the remaining marinade over the asparagus and let them marinate for 15-30 minutes.
4. Preheat your grill or grill pan to medium-high heat.

5. Thread the marinated shrimp onto skewers. If using wooden skewers, make sure they have been soaked in water to prevent burning.
6. Grill the shrimp skewers for 2-3 minutes per side, or until the shrimp are opaque and cooked through. Remove from the grill and set aside.
7. Grill the marinated asparagus spears for 3-4 minutes per side, or until tender and slightly charred.
8. Arrange the grilled shrimp and asparagus on plates and serve immediately. Enjoy your tasty Lemon Herb Grilled Shrimp and Asparagus dish!

Chicken Caprese Salad

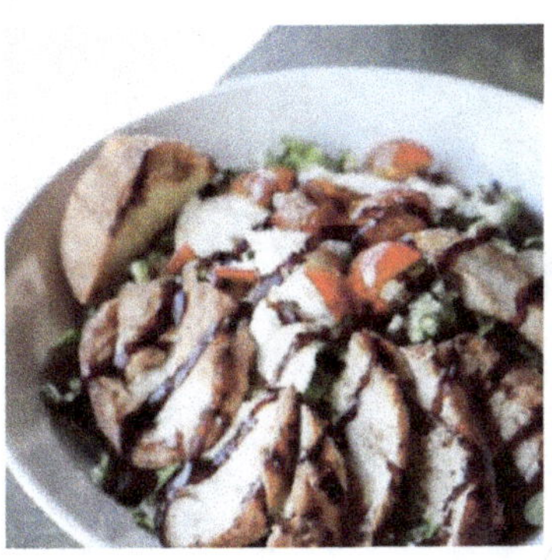

Portion Size: 4 servings

Macronutrient Breakdown (per serving):

- Calories: 380
- Protein: 42g
- Carbohydrates: 12g
- Fat: 18g
- Fibre: 3g

Ingredients:

- 4 boneless, skinless chicken breasts
- Salt and pepper, to taste
- 1 tablespoon olive oil
- 8 cups mixed greens
- 2 large ripe tomatoes, sliced
- 8 ounces fresh mozzarella cheese, sliced
- 1/2 cup fresh basil leaves
- 1/2 cup balsamic glaze

Instructions:

1. Season the chicken breasts with salt and pepper.
2. Heat olive oil in a grill pan or outdoor grill over medium-high heat. Grill the chicken breasts for 6-8 minutes per side, or until fully cooked and internal temperature reaches 165°F (74°C). Let the chicken rest for a few minutes, then slice it into strips.
3. On four individual plates, create a bed of mixed greens.
4. Arrange the sliced grilled chicken, tomato slices, and mozzarella slices on top of the greens, in a visually pleasing manner.
5. Scatter fresh basil leaves over the salad.
6. Drizzle the balsamic glaze over the Chicken Caprese Salad, ensuring each serving receives an equal amount.

7.   Serve immediately, and enjoy your delicious and healthy Chicken
      Caprese Salad!

Turkey Taco Stuffed Bell Peppers

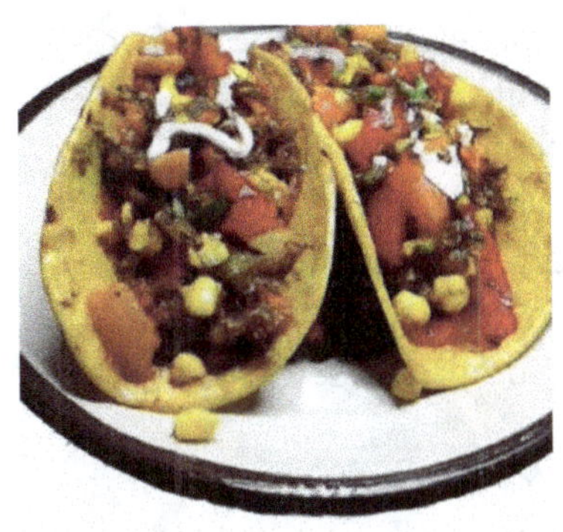

Portion Size: 4 servings (2 stuffed pepper halves per serving)

Macronutrient Breakdown (per serving):

- Calories: 410
- Protein: 34g
- Carbohydrates: 34g
- Fat: 16g
- Fibre: 7g

Ingredients:

- 4 bell peppers (assorted colours), halved and seeded
- 1 pound lean ground turkey
- 1 tablespoon olive oil
- 1 small onion, chopped
- 2 cloves garlic, minced
- 1 tablespoon taco seasoning
- 1/2 cup canned black beans, drained and rinsed
- 1/2 cup frozen corn, thawed
- Salt and pepper, to taste
- 1 cup shredded cheddar cheese
- Optional toppings: diced tomatoes, chopped cilantro, sour cream, sliced avocado

Instructions:

1. Preheat your oven to 375°F (190°C).
2. Heat olive oil in a large skillet over medium heat. Add the chopped onion and cook for 2-3 minutes until softened. Add garlic and cook for an additional 30 seconds.

3.   Add the ground turkey to the skillet, breaking it up with a spoon. Cook until the turkey is browned and fully cooked through. Drain any excess fat.
4.   Stir in the taco seasoning, black beans, corn, salt, and pepper. Cook for an additional 2-3 minutes, allowing the flavours to meld together.
5.   Place the halved bell peppers in a 9x13-inch baking dish, open-side up.
6.   Spoon the turkey taco mixture evenly into the bell pepper halves.
7.   Cover the baking dish with aluminium foil and bake for 30 minutes.
8.   Remove the foil and sprinkle shredded cheddar cheese evenly over the stuffed peppers.
9.   Return the peppers to the oven and bake for an additional 5-10 minutes, or until the cheese is melted and bubbly.
10.   Allow the stuffed peppers to cool for a few minutes before serving. Add optional toppings as desired, and enjoy your tasty Turkey Taco Stuffed Bell Peppers!

Baked Salmon with Lemon Dill Sauce

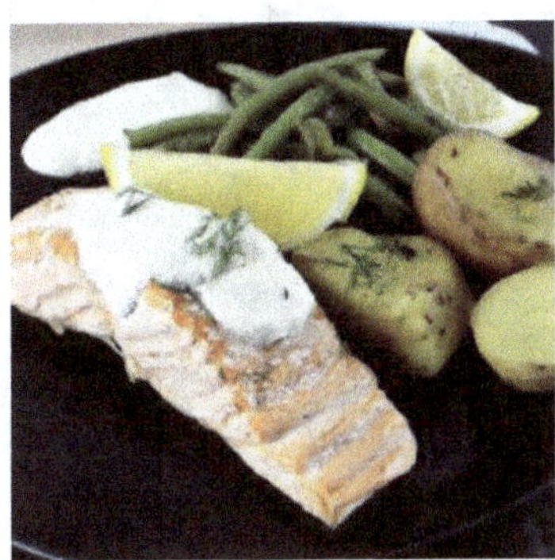

Portion Size: 4 servings

Macronutrient Breakdown (per serving):

- Calories: 410
- Protein: 36g
- Carbohydrates: 16g
- Fat: 22g
- Fibre: 4g

Ingredients:

- 4 salmon fillets (about 6 ounces each)
- Salt and pepper, to taste
- 1 tablespoon olive oil

Lemon Dill Sauce:

- 1/2 cup Greek yogurt or sour cream
- 2 tablespoons mayonnaise
- 1 tablespoon fresh lemon juice
- 1 tablespoon chopped fresh dill
- 1 teaspoon grated lemon zest
- 1 small garlic clove, minced
- Salt and pepper, to taste

Sides:

- 1 pound green beans, steamed
- 1 pound baby potatoes, roasted

Instructions:

1.   Preheat your oven to 400°F (200°C). Line a baking sheet with parchment paper.
2.   Pat the salmon fillets dry with paper towels, and season them with salt and pepper on both sides.
3.   Arrange the salmon fillets on the prepared baking sheet, skin-side down, and drizzle them with olive oil.
4.   Bake the salmon for 12-15 minutes, or until it flakes easily with a fork and reaches an internal temperature of 145°F (63°C).
5.   While the salmon bakes, prepare the lemon dill sauce by whisking together Greek yogurt or sour cream, mayonnaise, lemon juice, chopped dill, lemon zest, minced garlic, salt, and pepper in a small bowl. Taste and adjust the seasoning as needed.
6.   Plate the baked salmon fillets, and drizzle each fillet with a generous spoonful of the lemon dill sauce.
7.   Serve the salmon with steamed green beans and roasted baby potatoes on the side. Enjoy your delicious Baked Salmon with Lemon Dill Sauce!

Chicken Fajita Stuffed Spaghetti Squash

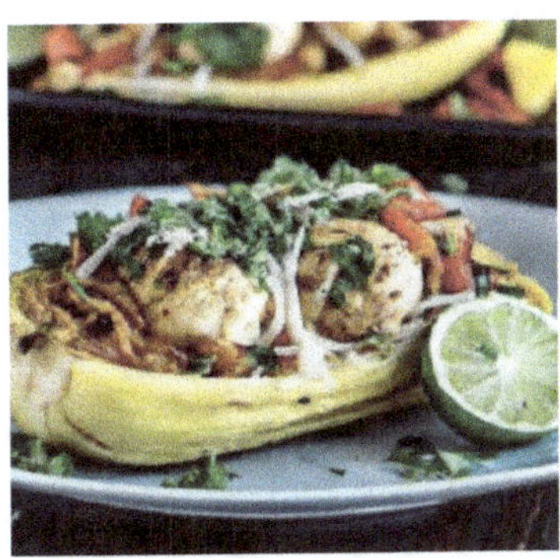

Portion Size: 4 servings

Macronutrient Breakdown (per serving):

- Calories: 410
- Protein: 38g
- Carbohydrates: 32g
- Fat: 16g
- Fibre: 7g

Ingredients:

- 2 medium spaghetti squash, halved and seeded
- 1 pound boneless, skinless chicken breast, cut into strips
- 1 tablespoon olive oil
- 1 small onion, thinly sliced
- 1 red bell pepper, thinly sliced
- 1 green bell pepper, thinly sliced
- 1 tablespoon fajita seasoning
- Salt and pepper, to taste
- Optional toppings: avocado, sour cream, chopped cilantro, lime wedges, shredded cheese

Instructions:

1. Preheat your oven to 400°F (200°C). Line a baking sheet with parchment paper.
2. Place the spaghetti squash halves cut-side down on the prepared baking sheet. Bake for 35-45 minutes, or until the squash is tender and can be easily shredded with a fork.
3. While the squash bakes, heat the olive oil in a large skillet over medium heat. Add the onion and bell peppers, and sauté until they are softened, about 5 minutes.

4.   Add the chicken strips to the skillet, and cook until they are no longer pink and cooked through. Stir in the fajita seasoning, salt, and pepper, and continue cooking for another 2-3 minutes.

5.   Remove the baked spaghetti squash from the oven, and carefully shred the inside with a fork to create spaghetti-like strands, leaving a thin layer of squash attached to the skin.

6.   Spoon the chicken fajita mixture into each spaghetti squash half, making sure it's evenly distributed.

7.   Return the stuffed spaghetti squash halves to the oven, and bake for an additional 10 minutes.

8.   Remove the stuffed squash from the oven and let them cool for a few minutes. Add optional toppings as desired, and serve immediately. Enjoy your scrumptious Chicken Fajita Stuffed Spaghetti Squash!

Quinoa, Beet, and Goat Cheese Salad

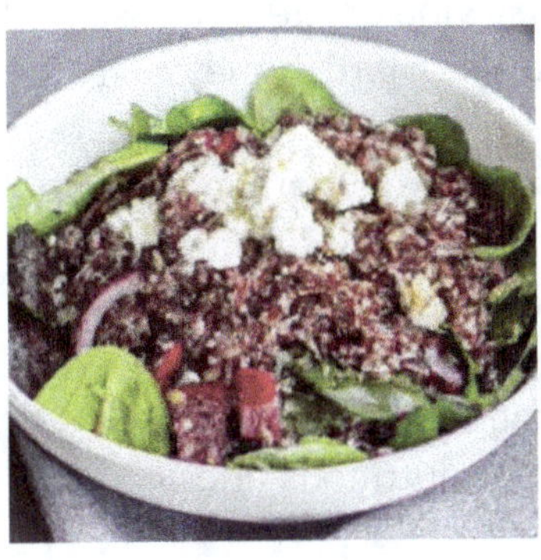

Portion Size: 4 servings

Macronutrient Breakdown (per serving):

- Calories: 420
- Protein: 15g
- Carbohydrates: 48g
- Fat: 20g
- Fibre: 7g

Ingredients:

- 1 cup uncooked quinoa
- 2 cups water
- 4 medium beets, roasted, peeled, and diced
- 4 cups baby spinach
- 1/2 cup crumbled goat cheese
- 1/2 cup chopped walnuts, toasted

Balsamic Vinaigrette:

- 1/4 cup balsamic vinegar
- 1/4 cup olive oil
- 1 tablespoon Dijon mustard
- 1 tablespoon honey
- Salt and pepper, to taste

Instructions:

1. In a medium saucepan, bring the water to a boil. Add the quinoa, reduce the heat to low, and cover the saucepan. Cook the quinoa for 15-20 minutes, or until the water is absorbed and the quinoa is

tender. Remove the saucepan from heat and let it stand for 5 minutes. Fluff the quinoa with a fork, and then let it cool.
2. While the quinoa cooks, prepare the balsamic vinaigrette by whisking together the balsamic vinegar, olive oil, Dijon mustard, honey, salt, and pepper in a small bowl.
3. In a large salad bowl, combine the cooked and cooled quinoa, roasted diced beets, baby spinach, crumbled goat cheese, and toasted chopped walnuts. Drizzle the balsamic vinaigrette over the salad, and gently toss to combine.
4. Serve the Quinoa, Beet, and Goat Cheese Salad immediately, or cover and refrigerate until ready to serve. Enjoy your nutritious and flavourful salad!

Turkey Meatball and Vegetable Stir Fry

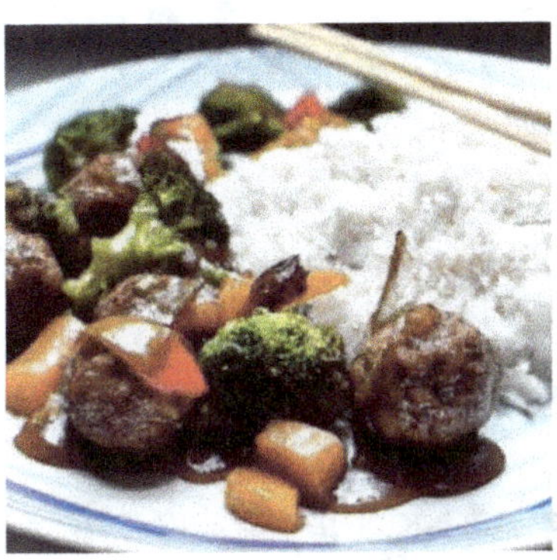

Portion Size: 4 servings

Macronutrient Breakdown (per serving):

- Calories: 450
- Protein: 32g
- Carbohydrates: 50g
- Fat: 15g
- Fibre: 6g

Ingredients:

- 1 pound ground turkey
- 1/4 cup breadcrumbs
- 1 large egg
- Salt and pepper, to taste

Stir Fry:

- 1 tablespoon vegetable oil
- 2 cups broccoli florets
- 1 red bell pepper, sliced
- 1 yellow bell pepper, sliced
- 1 cup sliced carrots

Sauce:

- 1/4 cup soy sauce
- 1/4 cup chicken broth
- 1 tablespoon hoisin sauce
- 1 tablespoon rice vinegar
- 2 teaspoons corn starch

- 1 teaspoon grated fresh ginger
- 2 cloves garlic, minced

For serving:

- Steamed brown rice

Instructions:

1. Preheat your oven to 400°F (200°C). Line a baking sheet with parchment paper.
2. In a large bowl, combine the ground turkey, breadcrumbs, egg, salt, and pepper. Mix until well combined.
3. Shape the turkey mixture into 1-inch meatballs and place them on the prepared baking sheet. Bake for 20-25 minutes, or until cooked through and golden brown.
4. While the meatballs bake, heat the vegetable oil in a large skillet or wok over medium-high heat. Add the broccoli, bell peppers, and carrots, and stir fry for 5-7 minutes, or until the vegetables are crisp-tender.
5. In a small bowl, whisk together the soy sauce, chicken broth, hoisin sauce, rice vinegar, corn starch, ginger, and garlic. Pour the sauce mixture over the stir-fried vegetables and cook for an additional 2-3 minutes, until the sauce has thickened.
6. Add the cooked turkey meatballs to the skillet and gently stir to coat them in the sauce.
7. Serve the Turkey Meatball and Vegetable Stir Fry over a bed of steamed brown rice. Enjoy your wholesome and satisfying meal!

Mediterranean Shrimp and Couscous Salad

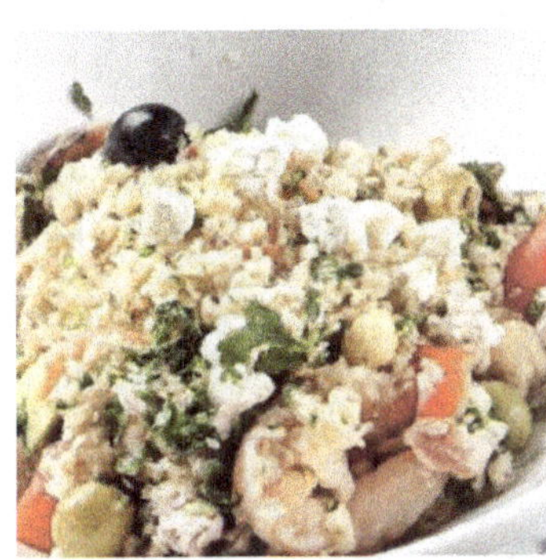

Portion Size: 4 servings

Macronutrient Breakdown (per serving):

- Calories: 450
- Protein: 28g
- Carbohydrates: 48g
- Fat: 17g
- Fibre: 5g

Ingredients:

- 1 cup uncooked couscous
- 1 1/4 cups water
- 1 pound cooked shrimp, peeled and deveined
- 1 cup cherry tomatoes, halved
- 1 cup diced cucumber
- 1/2 cup Kalamata olives, pitted and halved
- 1/2 cup crumbled feta cheese

Lemon Herb Dressing:

- 1/4 cup olive oil
- 1/4 cup fresh lemon juice
- 2 tablespoons chopped fresh parsley
- 1 tablespoon chopped fresh mint
- 1 small garlic clove, minced
- Salt and pepper, to taste

Instructions:

1. In a medium saucepan, bring the water to a boil. Add the couscous, cover the saucepan, and remove it from the heat. Let it stand for 5

minutes, until the water is absorbed and the couscous is tender. Fluff the couscous with a fork and let it cool.

2.   While the couscous cools, prepare the lemon herb dressing by whisking together the olive oil, lemon juice, parsley, mint, garlic, salt, and pepper in a small bowl.

3.   In a large salad bowl, combine the cooled couscous, cooked shrimp, cherry tomatoes, cucumber, Kalamata olives, and feta cheese. Drizzle the lemon herb dressing over the salad and gently toss to combine.

4.   Serve the Mediterranean Shrimp and Couscous Salad immediately, or cover and refrigerate until ready to serve. Enjoy this refreshing and flavourful salad!

Grilled Chicken and Pineapple Salsa Bowl

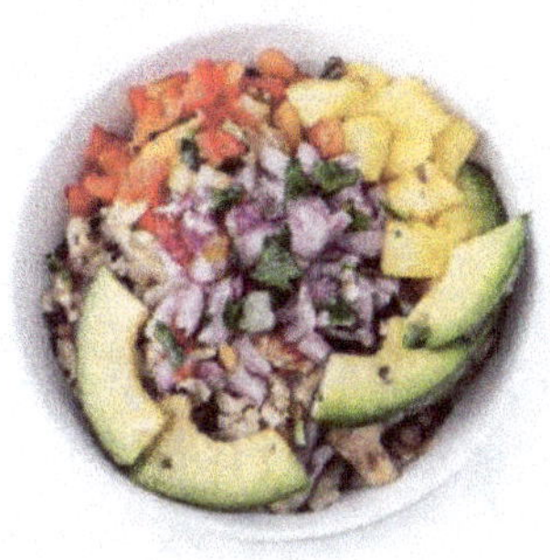

Portion Size: 4 servings

Macronutrient Breakdown (per serving):

- Calories: 460
- Protein: 38g
- Carbohydrates: 53g
- Fat: 12g
- Fibre: 8g

Ingredients:

- 4 boneless, skinless chicken breasts
- Salt and pepper, to taste

Marinade:

- 1/4 cup fresh lime juice
- 1/4 cup olive oil
- 2 cloves garlic, minced
- 1 teaspoon ground cumin
- Salt and pepper, to taste

Pineapple Salsa:

- 2 cups diced fresh pineapple
- 1/2 cup diced red onion
- 1/4 cup chopped fresh cilantro
- 1 jalapeño, seeded and minced
- Salt and pepper, to taste

Sides:

- 3 cups cooked brown rice
- 1 can (15 oz) black beans, drained and rinsed
- 2 avocados, sliced

Instructions:

1. In a small bowl, whisk together the lime juice, olive oil, garlic, cumin, salt, and pepper to create the marinade.
2. Place the chicken breasts in a shallow dish or a large resealable plastic bag, and pour the marinade over them. Refrigerate for at least 30 minutes, or up to 2 hours.
3. While the chicken marinates, prepare the pineapple salsa by combining the pineapple, red onion, cilantro, jalapeño, salt, and pepper in a medium bowl. Mix well and set aside.
4. Preheat your grill or a grill pan to medium-high heat. Remove the chicken from the marinade, discarding any excess marinade.
5. Grill the chicken for 5-7 minutes per side, or until it is cooked through and reaches an internal temperature of 165°F (74°C). Transfer the chicken to a plate and let it rest for 5 minutes before slicing.
6. Assemble the Grilled Chicken and Pineapple Salsa Bowls by dividing the cooked brown rice among four bowls. Top each bowl with sliced grilled chicken, a generous spoonful of pineapple salsa, black beans, and avocado slices.
7. Serve immediately, and enjoy your fresh and delicious Grilled Chicken and Pineapple Salsa Bowl!

Asian Salmon and Veggie Quinoa Bowl

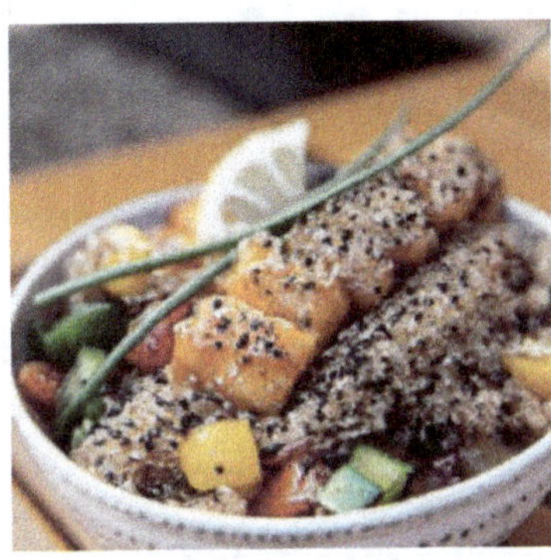

Portion Size: 4 servings

Macronutrient Breakdown (per serving):

- Calories: 465
- Protein: 36g
- Carbohydrates: 50g
- Fat: 15g
- Fibre: 8g

Ingredients:

- 4 salmon fillets (4-6 oz each)
- Salt and pepper, to taste

Sauce:

- 1/4 cup low-sodium soy sauce
- 2 tablespoons honey
- 2 tablespoons rice vinegar
- 1 tablespoon grated fresh ginger
- 2 cloves garlic, minced

Quinoa:

- 1 cup uncooked quinoa
- 2 cups water

Veggies:

- 1 tablespoon olive oil
- 1 red bell pepper, sliced
- 1 yellow bell pepper, sliced

- 2 cups broccoli florets
- 1 cup sliced carrots
- Salt and pepper, to taste

Toppings:

- Sesame seeds
- Sliced green onions

Instructions:

1. Preheat your oven to 400°F (200°C). Line a baking sheet with foil.
2. In a small saucepan, combine the soy sauce, honey, rice vinegar, ginger, and garlic. Cook over medium heat, stirring occasionally, until the sauce thickens slightly. Set aside.
3. Place the salmon fillets on the prepared baking sheet and season with salt and pepper. Brush the sauce generously over the salmon fillets. Bake for 12-15 minutes, or until the salmon is cooked through and flakes easily with a fork.
4. While the salmon bakes, bring the water to a boil in a medium saucepan. Add the quinoa, reduce the heat to low, and cover. Cook the quinoa for 15-20 minutes, or until the water is absorbed and the quinoa is tender. Remove from heat, fluff with a fork, and keep warm.
5. In a large skillet, heat the olive oil over medium-high heat. Add the bell peppers, broccoli, and carrots. Sauté for 5-7 minutes, or until the vegetables are tender-crisp. Season with salt and pepper.
6. Assemble the Asian Salmon and Veggie Quinoa Bowls by dividing the cooked quinoa among four bowls. Top each bowl with a salmon fillet and sautéed veggies. Drizzle any remaining sauce over the bowls.
7. Garnish the bowls with sesame seeds and sliced green onions. Serve immediately, and enjoy your flavourful and nutritious Asian Salmon and Veggie Quinoa Bowl!

Steak Fajita Zucchini Noodle Bowl

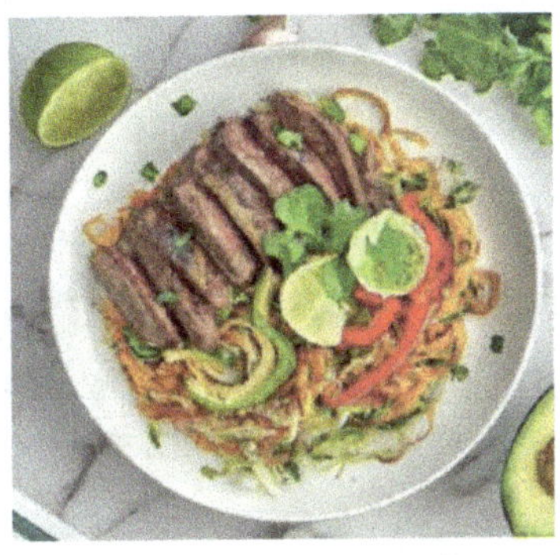

Portion Size: 4 servings

Macronutrient Breakdown (per serving):

- Calories: 450
- Protein: 35g
- Carbohydrates: 20g
- Fat: 25g
- Fibre: 6g

Ingredients:

- 1 pound flank steak, thinly sliced
- Salt and pepper, to taste

Fajita Marinade:

- 1/4 cup fresh lime juice
- 1/4 cup olive oil
- 1 teaspoon ground cumin
- 1 teaspoon chili powder
- 2 cloves garlic, minced
- Salt and pepper, to taste

Vegetables:

- 1 tablespoon olive oil
- 1 large red bell pepper, sliced
- 1 large green bell pepper, sliced
- 1 large onion, thinly sliced

Zucchini Noodles:

- 4 medium zucchinis, spiralized

Toppings:

- 1 avocado, diced
- Chopped cilantro
- Lime wedges

Instructions:

1. In a small bowl, whisk together the lime juice, olive oil, cumin, chili powder, garlic, salt, and pepper to create the fajita marinade.
2. Place the sliced steak in a shallow dish or a large resealable plastic bag, and pour the marinade over it. Refrigerate for at least 30 minutes, or up to 2 hours.
3. Heat 1 tablespoon of olive oil in a large skillet over medium-high heat. Add the bell peppers and onions, and cook for 5-7 minutes, or until they are tender and slightly charred. Remove the vegetables from the skillet and set them aside.
4. In the same skillet, cook the marinated steak for 3-4 minutes per side, or until it reaches your desired level of doneness. Transfer the cooked steak to a plate and let it rest for 5 minutes.
5. While the steak rests, sauté the spiralized zucchini noodles in the same skillet over medium heat for 2-3 minutes, or until they are tender. Be careful not to overcook them, as they can become mushy.
6. Assemble the Steak Fajita Zucchini Noodle Bowls by dividing the zucchini noodles among four bowls. Top each bowl with cooked steak, sautéed peppers and onions, and diced avocado.
7. Garnish the bowls with chopped cilantro and a squeeze of lime. Serve immediately, and enjoy your delicious and low-carb Steak Fajita Zucchini Noodle Bowl!

Chicken Caprese Salad Bowl

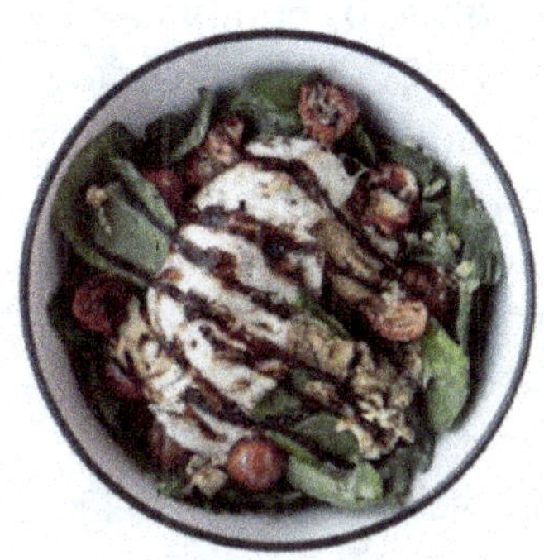

Portion Size: 4 servings

Macronutrient Breakdown (per serving):

- Calories: 380
- Protein: 35g
- Carbohydrates: 12g
- Fat: 22g
- Fibre: 3g

Ingredients:

- 4 boneless, skinless chicken breasts
- Salt and pepper, to taste

Caprese Salad:

- 2 cups mixed greens
- 1 cup cherry tomatoes, halved
- 1 cup fresh basil leaves
- 8 ounces fresh mozzarella cheese, sliced or cubed

Balsamic Glaze:

- 1/2 cup balsamic vinegar
- 2 tablespoons honey

Instructions:

1. Preheat your grill or grill pan to medium-high heat. Season the chicken breasts with salt and pepper. Grill the chicken for 5-7 minutes per side, or until cooked through and the internal temperature

reaches 165°F (74°C). Transfer the chicken to a plate and let it rest for 5 minutes before slicing.

2. While the chicken grills, prepare the balsamic glaze by combining the balsamic vinegar and honey in a small saucepan. Cook over medium heat, stirring occasionally, until the mixture is reduced by half and has a syrupy consistency. Remove from heat and let it cool slightly.

3. Assemble the Chicken Caprese Salad Bowls by dividing the mixed greens among four bowls. Top each bowl with sliced grilled chicken, cherry tomatoes, basil leaves, and mozzarella cheese.

4. Drizzle the balsamic glaze over each salad bowl, and serve immediately. Enjoy your fresh and flavourful Chicken Caprese Salad Bowl!

Spicy Shrimp and Vegetable Stir-Fry Bowl

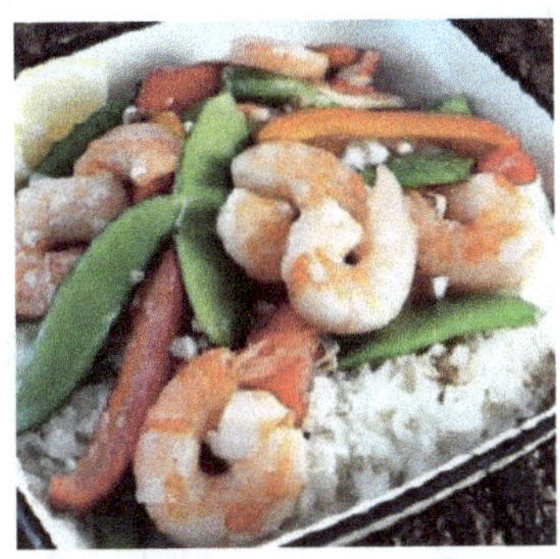

Portion Size: 4 servings

Macronutrient Breakdown (per serving):

- Calories: 410
- Protein: 30g
- Carbohydrates: 46g
- Fat: 12g
- Fibre: 5g

Ingredients:

- 1 pound large shrimp, peeled and deveined
- Salt and pepper, to taste

Stir-Fry Sauce:

- 1/4 cup low-sodium soy sauce
- 1/4 cup oyster sauce
- 2 tablespoons honey
- 2 tablespoons Sriracha (or to taste)
- 1 tablespoon corn starch
- 1/4 cup water

Vegetables:

- 1 tablespoon sesame oil
- 1 red bell pepper, sliced
- 1 cup snow peas
- 1 cup sliced carrots

Sides:

- 3 cups cooked white or brown rice

Toppings:

- Sliced green onions
- Sesame seeds

Instructions:

1. In a small bowl, whisk together the soy sauce, oyster sauce, honey, Sriracha, corn starch, and water to create the stir-fry sauce. Set aside.
2. Heat the sesame oil in a large skillet or wok over medium-high heat. Add the shrimp to the skillet and cook for 1-2 minutes per side, or until they are opaque and cooked through. Transfer the shrimp to a plate and set them aside.
3. In the same skillet, add the red bell pepper, snow peas, and carrots. Stir-fry the vegetables for 3-4 minutes, or until they are tender-crisp.
4. Return the cooked shrimp to the skillet and pour in the prepared stir-fry sauce. Stir to combine and cook for an additional 2-3 minutes, or until the sauce has thickened and the shrimp and vegetables are well-coated.
5. Assemble the Spicy Shrimp and Vegetable Stir-Fry Bowls by dividing the cooked rice among four bowls. Top each bowl with the shrimp and vegetable mixture.
6. Garnish the bowls with sliced green onions and a sprinkle of sesame seeds. Serve immediately, and enjoy your delicious and nutritious Spicy Shrimp and Vegetable Stir-Fry Bowl!

Greek Chicken Grain Bowl

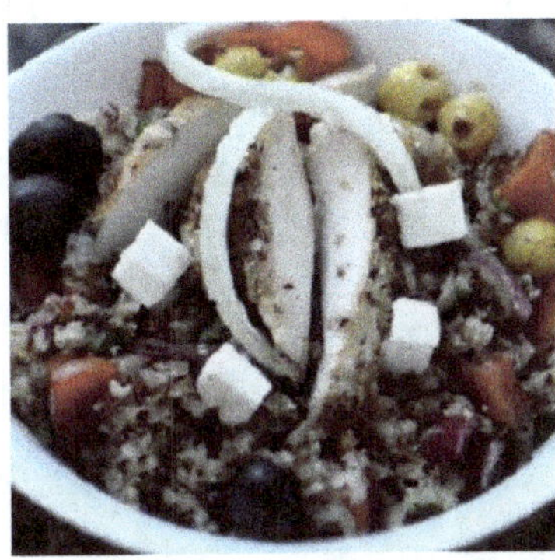

Portion Size: 4 servings

Macronutrient Breakdown (per serving):

- Calories: 480
- Protein: 32g
- Carbohydrates: 54g
- Fat: 17g
- Fibre: 8g

Ingredients:

- 4 boneless, skinless chicken breasts
- Salt and pepper, to taste

Marinade:

- 1/4 cup olive oil
- 1/4 cup lemon juice
- 2 cloves garlic, minced
- 1 teaspoon dried oregano
- Salt and pepper, to taste

Grain Base:

- 2 cups cooked farro or quinoa

Vegetables:

- 1 cup cherry tomatoes, halved
- 1 cup diced cucumber
- 1/2 cup diced red onion

Toppings:

- 1/2 cup pitted Kalamata olives, halved
- 1/2 cup crumbled feta cheese

Garnish:

- Fresh parsley, chopped

Instructions:

1. In a small bowl, whisk together the olive oil, lemon juice, garlic, oregano, salt, and pepper to create the marinade.
2. Place the chicken breasts in a shallow dish or a large resealable plastic bag, and pour the marinade over them. Refrigerate for at least 30 minutes, or up to 2 hours.
3. Preheat your grill or grill pan to medium-high heat. Remove the chicken breasts from the marinade and season with additional salt and pepper, if desired. Grill the chicken for 5-7 minutes per side, or until cooked through and the internal temperature reaches 165°F (74°C). Transfer the chicken to a plate and let it rest for 5 minutes before slicing.
4. Assemble the Greek Chicken Grain Bowls by dividing the cooked farro or quinoa among four bowls. Top each bowl with sliced grilled chicken, cherry tomatoes, cucumber, red onion, Kalamata olives, and crumbled feta cheese.
5. Garnish the bowls with chopped fresh parsley. Serve immediately, and enjoy your nutritious and flavourful Greek Chicken Grain Bowl!

Black Bean and Sweet Potato Burrito Bowl

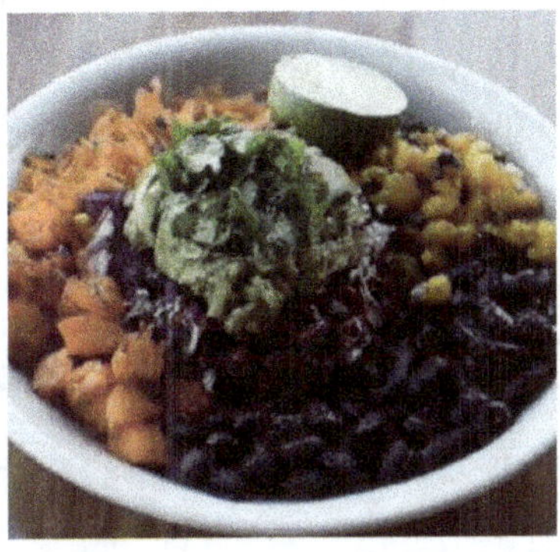

Portion Size: 4 servings

Macronutrient Breakdown (per serving):

- Calories: 500
- Protein: 16g
- Carbohydrates: 80g
- Fat: 15g
- Fibre: 15g

Ingredients:

- 2 medium sweet potatoes, peeled and diced
- 2 tablespoons olive oil
- 1 teaspoon ground cumin
- 1 teaspoon smoked paprika
- Salt and pepper, to taste

Base:

- 3 cups cooked brown rice or cauliflower rice

Toppings:

- 1 can (15 ounces) black beans, drained and rinsed
- 1 cup frozen charred corn, thawed
- 1 avocado, diced
- Lime wedges
- Fresh cilantro, chopped

Instructions:

1.   Preheat your oven to 400°F (200°C). In a large bowl, toss the diced sweet potatoes with olive oil, cumin, smoked paprika, salt, and pepper until evenly coated.
2.   Spread the seasoned sweet potatoes onto a lined baking sheet in a single layer. Roast in the oven for 25-30 minutes, or until they are tender and slightly caramelized.
3.   While the sweet potatoes are roasting, prepare the brown rice or cauliflower rice according to package instructions. Keep warm.
4.   Assemble the Black Bean and Sweet Potato Burrito Bowls by dividing the warm brown rice or cauliflower rice among four bowls. Top each bowl with roasted sweet potatoes, black beans, charred corn, and diced avocado.
5.   Squeeze lime wedges over each bowl and garnish with fresh cilantro. Serve immediately, and enjoy your healthy and satisfying Black Bean and Sweet Potato Burrito Bowl!

Salmon and Quinoa Salad Bowl

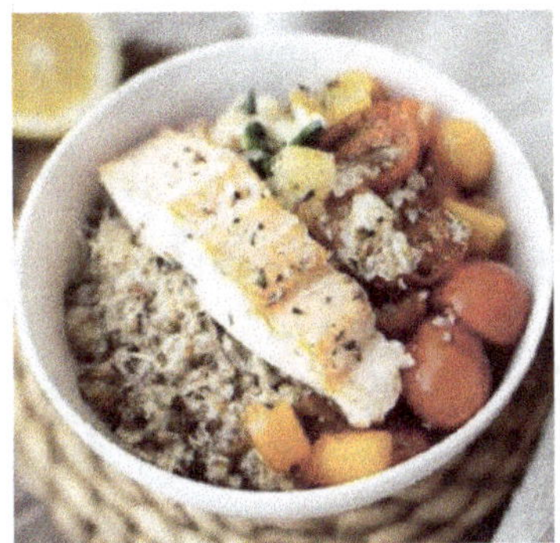

Portion Size: 4 servings

Macronutrient Breakdown (per serving):

- Calories: 470
- Protein: 38g
- Carbohydrates: 40g
- Fat: 19g
- Fibre: 6g

Ingredients:

- 4 salmon fillets (about 6 ounces each)
- Salt and pepper, to taste

Quinoa Salad:

- 2 cups cooked quinoa, cooled
- 2 cups baby spinach
- 1 cup roasted cherry tomatoes
- 1 cup diced cucumber

Lemon Vinaigrette:

- 1/4 cup olive oil
- 1/4 cup fresh lemon juice
- 1 clove garlic, minced
- Salt and pepper, to taste

Toppings:

- 1/2 cup crumbled feta cheese

Garnish:

- Fresh dill, chopped

Instructions:

1. Preheat your grill or grill pan to medium-high heat. Season the salmon fillets with salt and pepper. Grill the salmon for 4-5 minutes per side, or until cooked through and the internal temperature reaches 145°F (63°C). Transfer the salmon to a plate and let it rest for a few minutes.
2. In a large bowl, combine the cooled quinoa, baby spinach, roasted cherry tomatoes, and diced cucumber.
3. Prepare the lemon vinaigrette by whisking together the olive oil, lemon juice, minced garlic, salt, and pepper in a small bowl.
4. Pour the lemon vinaigrette over the quinoa salad and toss to combine.
5. Assemble the Salmon and Quinoa Salad Bowls by dividing the quinoa salad among four bowls. Top each bowl with a grilled salmon fillet and crumbled feta cheese.
6. Garnish the bowls with chopped fresh dill. Serve immediately, and enjoy your nutritious and delicious Salmon and Quinoa Salad Bowl!

Turkey Taco Stuffed Bell Pepper Bowl

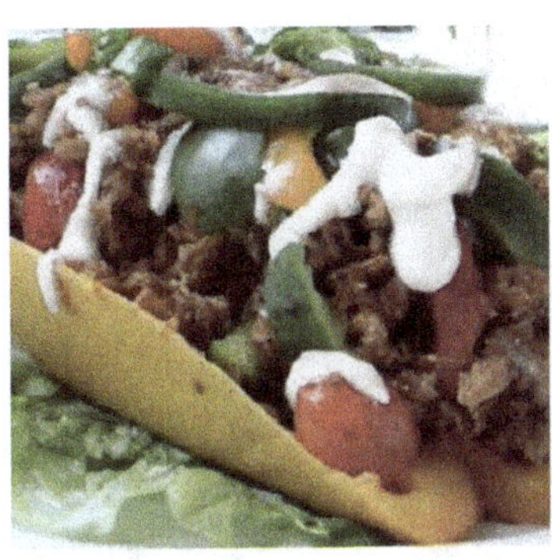

Portion Size: 4 servings

Macronutrient Breakdown (per serving):

- Calories: 460
- Protein: 35g
- Carbohydrates: 28g
- Fat: 23g
- Fibre: 9g

Ingredients:

- 4 large bell peppers (any colour), halved and seeds removed
- 1 tablespoon olive oil
- 1 pound lean ground turkey
- 1 small onion, diced
- 1 can (15 ounces) black beans, drained and rinsed
- 2 tablespoons taco seasoning

Base:

- 4 cups chopped romaine lettuce

Toppings:

- 1 avocado, sliced
- 1 cup non-fat Greek yogurt
- 1 cup shredded cheddar cheese

Instructions:

1. Preheat your oven to 375°F (190°C). Place the halved bell peppers cut-side up in a large baking dish.

2. Heat the olive oil in a large skillet over medium-high heat. Add the ground turkey and diced onion, and cook until the turkey is browned and cooked through. Drain any excess fat.

3. Stir in the black beans and taco seasoning, and cook for an additional 2-3 minutes, or until the mixture is heated through and well-combined.

4. Spoon the turkey taco mixture into the bell pepper halves, filling them evenly.

5. Cover the baking dish with aluminium foil, and bake the stuffed bell peppers for 25-30 minutes, or until the bell peppers are tender.

6. Assemble the Turkey Taco Stuffed Bell Pepper Bowls by placing a bed of chopped romaine lettuce in each bowl. Add a stuffed bell pepper half (or two, if desired) to each bowl.

7. Top each bowl with sliced avocado, a dollop of Greek yogurt, and a sprinkle of shredded cheddar cheese. Serve immediately, and enjoy your healthy and flavourful Turkey Taco Stuffed Bell Pepper Bowl!

Chicken Pesto Zucchini Noodle Bowl

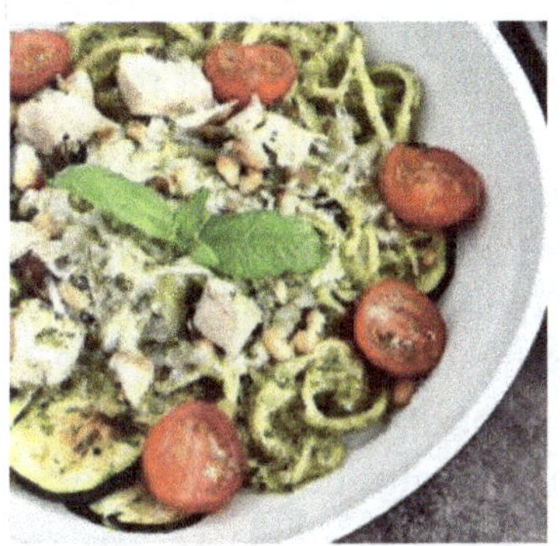

Portion Size: 4 servings

Macronutrient Breakdown (per serving):

- Calories: 430
- Protein: 34g
- Carbohydrates: 18g
- Fat: 27g
- Fibre: 5g

Ingredients:

- 4 boneless, skinless chicken breasts
- Salt and pepper, to taste
- 4 medium zucchini, spiralized
- 1 cup cherry tomatoes, halved
- 1/2 cup pitted Kalamata olives, halved

Pesto Sauce:

- 2 cups fresh basil leaves, packed
- 1/2 cup grated Parmesan cheese
- 1/3 cup toasted pine nuts
- 2 cloves garlic, minced
- 1/2 cup olive oil
- Salt and pepper, to taste

Garnish:

- Grated Parmesan cheese
- Toasted pine nuts

Instructions:

1. Preheat your grill or grill pan to medium-high heat. Season the chicken breasts with salt and pepper. Grill the chicken for 5-7 minutes per side, or until cooked through and the internal temperature reaches 165°F (74°C). Transfer the chicken to a plate and let it rest for a few minutes before slicing.
2. Prepare the pesto sauce by combining the basil, Parmesan cheese, toasted pine nuts, and minced garlic in a food processor. While the food processor is running, slowly drizzle in the olive oil until a smooth sauce forms. Season with salt and pepper to taste.
3. In a large bowl, toss the spiralized zucchini noodles, sliced grilled chicken, cherry tomatoes, and Kalamata olives with the homemade pesto sauce until well coated.
4. Assemble the Chicken Pesto Zucchini Noodle Bowls by dividing the mixture among four bowls.
5. Garnish the bowls with a sprinkle of grated Parmesan cheese and a few toasted pine nuts. Serve immediately, and enjoy your nutritious and delicious Chicken Pesto Zucchini Noodle Bowl!

Spicy Shrimp Cauliflower Fried Rice Bowl

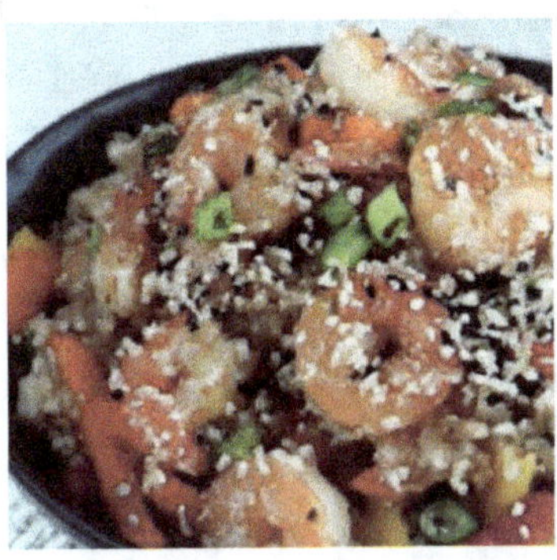

Portion Size: 4 servings

Macronutrient Breakdown (per serving):

- Calories: 350
- Protein: 26g
- Carbohydrates: 18g
- Fat: 19g
- Fibre: 6g

Ingredients:

- 1 pound large shrimp, peeled and deveined
- 2 tablespoons olive oil
- 2 cloves garlic, minced
- 1/4 teaspoon red pepper flakes
- Salt and pepper, to taste
- 1 small head cauliflower, riced (about 4 cups)
- 1/2 cup diced bell peppers (any colour)
- 1/2 cup frozen peas, thawed
- 2 tablespoons soy sauce
- 1 tablespoon sesame oil

Garnish:

- Chopped green onions
- Sesame seeds

Instructions:

1. In a large skillet, heat 1 tablespoon of olive oil over medium-high heat. Add the shrimp, garlic, and red pepper flakes, and season with

salt and pepper. Cook for 2-3 minutes per side, or until the shrimp are pink and cooked through. Transfer the shrimp to a plate and set aside.

2. In the same skillet, heat the remaining 1 tablespoon of olive oil over medium-high heat. Add the cauliflower rice, diced bell peppers, and thawed peas, stirring occasionally until the vegetables are tender, about 5-6 minutes.

3. Stir in the soy sauce and sesame oil, and cook for an additional 2 minutes, allowing the flavours to meld.

4. Return the cooked shrimp to the skillet and mix with the cauliflower fried rice, cooking for another 1-2 minutes until heated through.

5. Assemble the Spicy Shrimp Cauliflower Fried Rice Bowls by dividing the mixture among four bowls.

6. Garnish the bowls with chopped green onions and a sprinkle of sesame seeds. Serve immediately, and enjoy your nutritious and delicious Spicy Shrimp Cauliflower Fried Rice Bowl!

Beef and Broccoli Stir-Fry Bowl

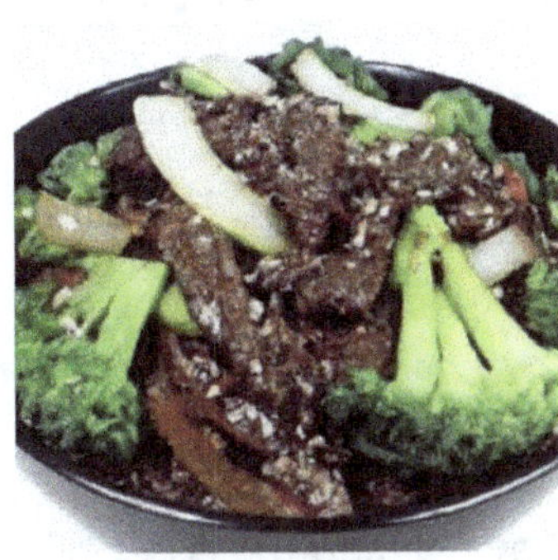

Portion Size: 4 servings

Macronutrient Breakdown (per serving):

- Calories: 450
- Protein: 34g
- Carbohydrates: 45g
- Fat: 15g
- Fibre: 5g

Ingredients:

- 1 pound flank steak, thinly sliced against the grain
- 2 tablespoons vegetable oil, divided
- 2 cloves garlic, minced
- 1 tablespoon fresh ginger, minced
- 1/4 cup soy sauce
- 1/4 cup oyster sauce
- 1/4 cup water
- 4 cups broccoli florets

Base:

- 4 cups cooked white or brown rice

Garnish:

- Thinly sliced green onions
- Sesame seeds

Instructions:

1.	In a large skillet or wok, heat 1 tablespoon of vegetable oil over medium-high heat. Add the sliced flank steak and cook for 3-4 minutes until browned on all sides. Transfer the beef to a plate and set aside.

2.	In the same skillet, heat the remaining 1 tablespoon of vegetable oil. Add the garlic and ginger, and cook for 1 minute until fragrant.

3.	Stir in the soy sauce, oyster sauce, and water, then add the broccoli florets. Cook for 3-4 minutes, stirring occasionally until the broccoli is tender-crisp.

4.	Return the cooked beef to the skillet and stir to combine, allowing the flavours to meld for an additional 2-3 minutes.

5.	Assemble the Beef and Broccoli Stir-Fry Bowls by dividing the cooked white or brown rice among four bowls. Top each bowl with the beef and broccoli mixture.

6.	Garnish the bowls with thinly sliced green onions and a sprinkle of sesame seeds. Serve immediately, and enjoy your flavourful and satisfying Beef and Broccoli Stir-Fry Bowl!

Chicken Fajita Stuffed Sweet Potato Bowl

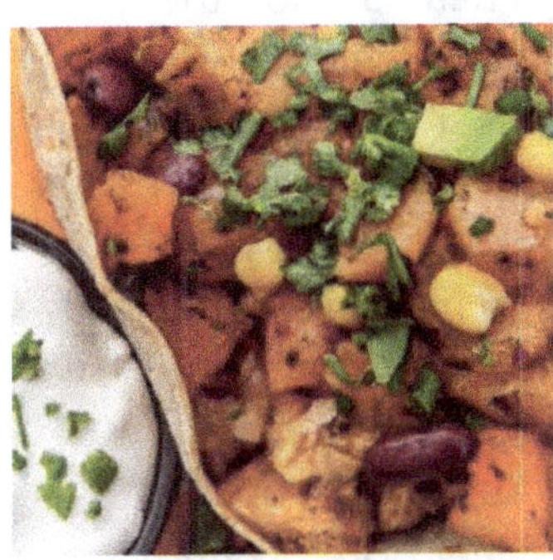

Portion Size: 4 servings

Macronutrient Breakdown (per serving):

- Calories: 490
- Protein: 34g
- Carbohydrates: 54g
- Fat: 17g
- Fibre: 11g

Ingredients:

- 4 medium sweet potatoes
- 1 pound boneless, skinless chicken breasts
- Salt and pepper, to taste
- 1 tablespoon olive oil
- 1 small onion, thinly sliced
- 1 red bell pepper, thinly sliced
- 1 yellow bell pepper, thinly sliced
- 2 tablespoons fajita seasoning

Toppings:

- 1 cup guacamole
- 1 cup pico de gallo
- 1/2 cup sour cream

Instructions:

1. Preheat your oven to 400°F (200°C). Wash and dry the sweet potatoes, then pierce each sweet potato several times with a fork. Wrap each sweet potato individually in aluminium foil, and place them on a baking sheet. Bake for 45-50 minutes, or until the sweet potatoes are

tender when pierced with a fork. Allow the sweet potatoes to cool slightly, then carefully slice them open and fluff the insides with a fork.

2. Preheat your grill or grill pan to medium-high heat. Season the chicken breasts with salt and pepper. Grill the chicken for 5-7 minutes per side, or until cooked through and the internal temperature reaches 165°F (74°C). Transfer the chicken to a plate and let it rest for a few minutes before slicing.

3. In a large skillet, heat the olive oil over medium heat. Add the sliced onion and bell peppers, and cook for 4-5 minutes until softened. Stir in the fajita seasoning and cook for an additional 1-2 minutes.

4. Assemble the Chicken Fajita Stuffed Sweet Potato Bowls by placing a baked sweet potato in each bowl. Top each sweet potato with the grilled chicken, sautéed bell peppers, and onions.

5. Add a generous spoonful of guacamole and pico de gallo to each bowl, and drizzle with sour cream. Serve immediately, and enjoy your tasty and nutritious Chicken Fajita Stuffed Sweet Potato Bowl!

Greek-Style Baked Cod Bowl

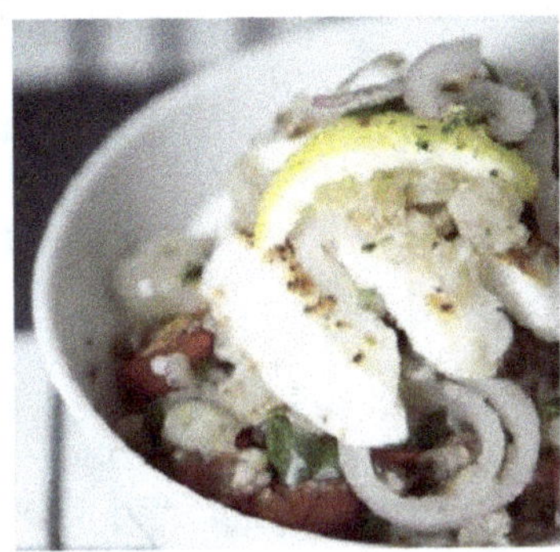

Portion Size: 4 servings

Macronutrient Breakdown (per serving):

- Calories: 470
- Protein: 40g
- Carbohydrates: 40g
- Fat: 16g
- Fibre: 7g

Ingredients:

- 4 (6-ounce) cod fillets
- 2 tablespoons olive oil
- 2 cloves garlic, minced
- Juice of 1 lemon
- 1 tablespoon dried oregano
- 1 teaspoon dried thyme
- Salt and pepper, to taste
- 4 cups cooked quinoa, warm

Cucumber-Tomato Salad:

- 1 large cucumber, diced
- 1 cup cherry tomatoes, halved
- 1/4 cup diced red onion
- 1/4 cup chopped fresh parsley
- 1 tablespoon olive oil
- Juice of 1 lemon
- Salt and pepper, to taste

Tzatziki Sauce:

- 1 cup Greek yogurt
- 1/2 cup grated cucumber, squeezed to remove excess liquid
- 1 clove garlic, minced
- 1 tablespoon fresh dill, chopped
- Juice of 1/2 lemon
- Salt and pepper, to taste

Instructions:

1. Preheat your oven to 400°F (200°C). In a small bowl, whisk together the olive oil, minced garlic, lemon juice, oregano, thyme, salt, and pepper. Place the cod fillets in a baking dish, and pour the marinade over the top. Allow the fillets to marinate for 15 minutes.
2. Bake the marinated cod fillets for 12-15 minutes, or until the fish flakes easily with a fork.
3. Meanwhile, prepare the cucumber-tomato salad by combining the cucumber, cherry tomatoes, red onion, parsley, olive oil, and lemon juice in a bowl. Season with salt and pepper, to taste.
4. In a separate bowl, prepare the tzatziki sauce by combining the Greek yogurt, grated cucumber, minced garlic, fresh dill, and lemon juice. Season with salt and pepper, to taste.
5. Assemble the Greek-Style Baked Cod Bowls by placing a bed of warm quinoa in each bowl. Top each bowl with a baked cod fillet, a generous spoonful of cucumber-tomato salad, and a dollop of tzatziki sauce. Serve immediately, and enjoy your wholesome and delectable Greek-Style Baked Cod Bowl!

Turkey and Veggie Stir-Fry Bowl

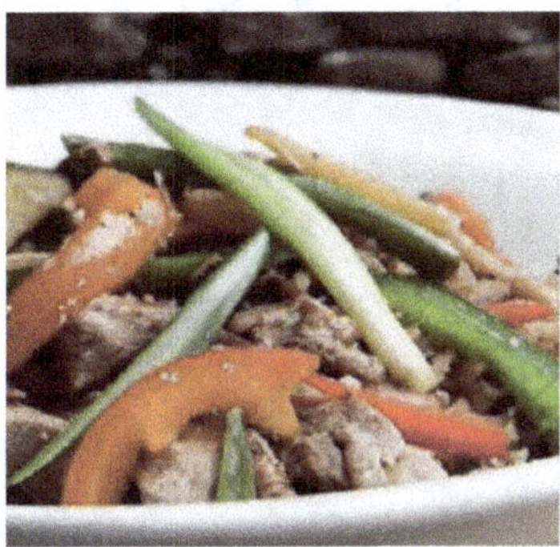

Portion Size: 4 servings

Macronutrient Breakdown (per serving):

- Calories: 480
- Protein: 36g
- Carbohydrates: 55g
- Fat: 14g
- Fibre: 8g

Ingredients:

- 1 pound ground turkey
- 1 tablespoon vegetable oil
- 2 cloves garlic, minced
- 1 tablespoon fresh ginger, minced
- 1/2 cup julienned carrots
- 1 red bell pepper, sliced
- 1 yellow bell pepper, sliced
- 1 cup snap peas
- 1/4 cup soy sauce
- 1 tablespoon sesame oil

Base:

- 4 cups cooked brown rice

Garnish:

- Sliced green onions
- Sesame seeds

Instructions:

1. In a large skillet or wok, heat the vegetable oil over medium-high heat. Add the ground turkey, garlic, and ginger, and cook for 5-7 minutes, breaking up the turkey as it cooks, until it is cooked through and no longer pink. Transfer the cooked turkey to a plate and set aside.

2. In the same skillet, add the julienned carrots, sliced bell peppers, and snap peas. Cook for 4-5 minutes, stirring occasionally, until the vegetables are tender-crisp.

3. Return the cooked turkey to the skillet, and stir in the soy sauce and sesame oil. Cook for an additional 2-3 minutes, allowing the flavours to meld.

4. Assemble the Turkey and Veggie Stir-Fry Bowls by dividing the cooked brown rice among four bowls. Top each bowl with the turkey and vegetable mixture.

5. Garnish the bowls with sliced green onions and a sprinkle of sesame seeds. Serve immediately, and enjoy your nutritious and delicious Turkey and Veggie Stir-Fry Bowl!

Shrimp, Mango, and Avocado Quinoa Salad

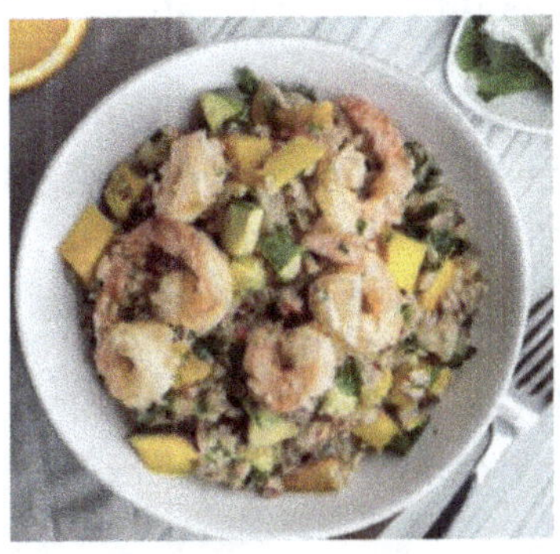

Portion Size: 4 servings

Macronutrient Breakdown (per serving):

- Calories: 465
- Protein: 30g
- Carbohydrates: 50g
- Fat: 18g
- Fibre: 9g

Ingredients:

- 1 pound large shrimp, peeled and deveined
- 2 tablespoons olive oil
- Salt and pepper, to taste
- 2 cups cooked quinoa, cooled
- 1 ripe mango, peeled and diced
- 1 large avocado, sliced
- 1 red bell pepper, diced
- 1/4 cup fresh cilantro, chopped

Lime Vinaigrette:

- 1/4 cup fresh lime juice
- 1/4 cup olive oil
- 2 teaspoons honey
- 1 clove garlic, minced
- Salt and pepper, to taste

Instructions:

1. Preheat your grill or grill pan to medium-high heat. Toss the shrimp in 2 tablespoons of olive oil and season with salt and pepper. Grill the

shrimp for 2-3 minutes per side, or until cooked through and opaque. Set the cooked shrimp aside to cool slightly.

2. In a large mixing bowl, combine the cooked quinoa, diced mango, sliced avocado, diced bell pepper, and chopped cilantro.

3. In a small bowl or jar, whisk together the fresh lime juice, olive oil, honey, minced garlic, salt, and pepper to create the lime vinaigrette.

4. Pour the lime vinaigrette over the quinoa mixture and gently toss to coat. Add the grilled shrimp to the salad and toss once more.

5. Divide the Shrimp, Mango, and Avocado Quinoa Salad among four bowls. Serve immediately or refrigerate until ready to serve. Enjoy your refreshing and protein-packed Shrimp, Mango, and Avocado Quinoa Salad!

Beef and Broccoli Quinoa Bowl

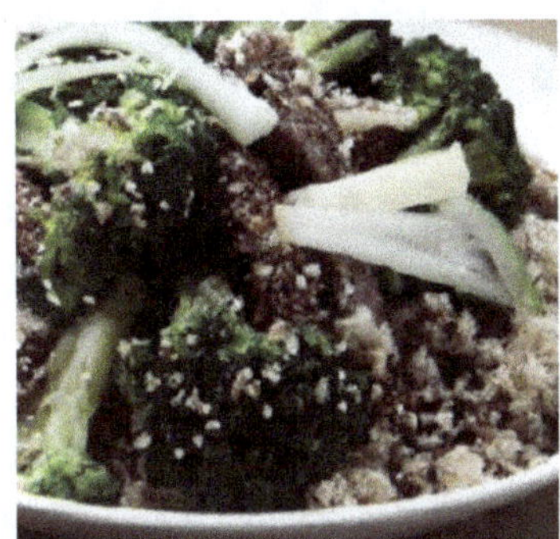

Portion Size: 4 servings

Macronutrient Breakdown (per serving):

- Calories: 475
- Protein: 34g
- Carbohydrates: 52g
- Fat: 17g
- Fibre: 7g

Ingredients:

- 1 pound flank steak, thinly sliced
- 4 cups broccoli florets
- 2 tablespoons vegetable oil
- 2 cloves garlic, minced
- 4 cups cooked quinoa

Marinade:

- 1/4 cup soy sauce
- 1 tablespoon corn starch
- 1 tablespoon hoisin sauce
- 1 tablespoon rice vinegar
- 1/2 teaspoon crushed red pepper flakes

Garnish:

- Chopped green onions
- Toasted sesame seeds

Instructions:

1. In a small bowl, whisk together the soy sauce, corn starch, hoisin sauce, rice vinegar, and crushed red pepper flakes. Add the thinly sliced flank steak to the marinade, making sure all the pieces are well coated. Cover and refrigerate for at least 30 minutes.

2. In a large skillet or wok, heat 1 tablespoon of vegetable oil over medium-high heat. Add the broccoli florets and cook for 4-5 minutes, or until tender-crisp. Transfer the cooked broccoli to a plate and set aside.

3. In the same skillet, heat another tablespoon of vegetable oil over medium-high heat. Add the minced garlic and sauté for about 30 seconds, or until fragrant. Add the marinated beef, discarding any remaining marinade, and stir-fry for 3-4 minutes, or until the beef is cooked through.

4. Return the cooked broccoli to the skillet, and stir-fry for an additional 2 minutes, until the beef and broccoli are heated through and well combined.

5. Assemble the Beef and Broccoli Quinoa Bowls by dividing the cooked quinoa among four bowls. Top each bowl with an even portion of the beef and broccoli mixture.

6. Garnish the bowls with chopped green onions and a sprinkle of toasted sesame seeds. Serve immediately, and enjoy your satisfying and nourishing Beef and Broccoli Quinoa Bowl!

Spinach and Feta Stuffed Chicken Breast

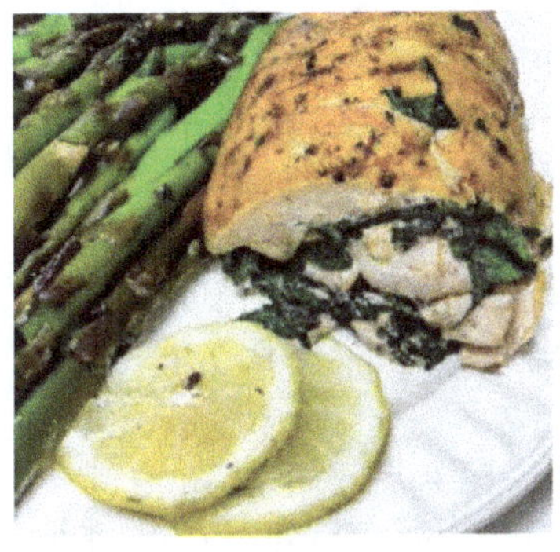

Portion Size: 4 servings

Macronutrient Breakdown (per serving):

- Calories: 410
- Protein: 43g
- Carbohydrates: 12g
- Fat: 20g
- Fibre: 4g

Ingredients:

- 4 boneless, skinless chicken breasts
- 1 tablespoon olive oil
- 1 small onion, finely chopped
- 2 cloves garlic, minced
- 4 cups baby spinach
- 1 cup crumbled feta cheese
- Salt and pepper, to taste

Lemony Roasted Asparagus:

- 1 pound fresh asparagus, trimmed
- 2 tablespoons olive oil
- Juice of 1 lemon
- Salt and pepper, to taste

Instructions:

1. Preheat your oven to 375°F (190°C). In a large skillet, heat 1 tablespoon of olive oil over medium heat. Add the chopped onion and minced garlic, and sauté for 4-5 minutes, or until the onions are soft and translucent.

2. Add the baby spinach to the skillet, and cook for 2-3 minutes, or until the spinach has wilted. Remove the skillet from the heat and stir in the crumbled feta cheese. Season with salt and pepper, to taste.

3. Use a sharp knife to create a deep pocket in each chicken breast, being careful not to cut all the way through. Stuff each pocket with the spinach and feta mixture, and secure the chicken breasts with toothpicks if needed.

4. Place the stuffed chicken breasts in a lightly greased baking dish, and bake for 25-30 minutes, or until the chicken is cooked through and no longer pink in the centre.

5. Meanwhile, prepare the lemony roasted asparagus by arranging the trimmed asparagus on a baking sheet. Drizzle the asparagus with olive oil and lemon juice, and season with salt and pepper, to taste. Roast the asparagus in the oven for 12-15 minutes, or until tender-crisp.

6. To serve, place a spinach and feta stuffed chicken breast on each plate, along with a side of lemony roasted asparagus. Enjoy your wholesome and mouth-watering Spinach and Feta Stuffed Chicken Breast!

Lentil and Sweet Potato Curry

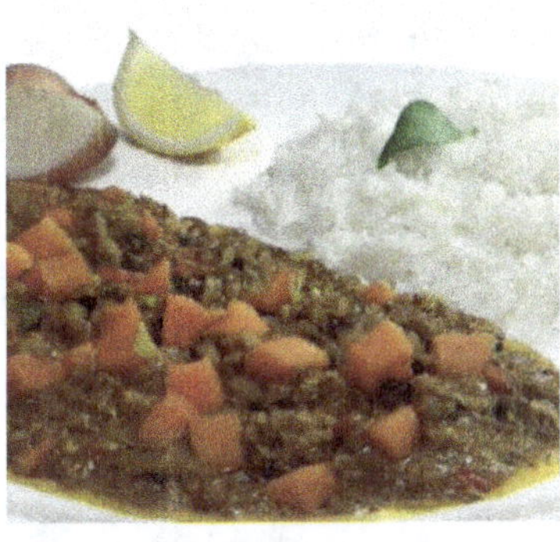

Portion Size: 4 servings

Macronutrient Breakdown (per serving):

- Calories: 435
- Protein: 18g
- Carbohydrates: 68g
- Fat: 10g
- Fibre: 15g

Ingredients:

- 1 cup dry green lentils, rinsed and drained
- 1 tablespoon vegetable oil
- 1 medium onion, chopped
- 2 cloves garlic, minced
- 1 tablespoon fresh ginger, minced
- 2 cups diced sweet potatoes
- 1 red bell pepper, chopped
- 1 tablespoon curry powder
- 1 teaspoon ground cumin
- 1/4 teaspoon cayenne pepper (optional)
- 1 (14-ounce) can coconut milk
- 2 cups vegetable broth
- Salt and pepper, to taste

For serving:

- 4 cups cooked basmati rice

Instructions:

1. In a medium saucepan, add the green lentils and cover with water. Bring to a boil, reduce heat, and simmer for 20-25 minutes or until lentils are tender but not mushy. Drain and set aside.
2. In a large pot, heat the vegetable oil over medium heat. Add the chopped onion, minced garlic, and fresh ginger, and sauté for 5-6 minutes, or until the onions are soft and translucent.
3. Add the diced sweet potatoes, chopped bell pepper, curry powder, ground cumin, and cayenne pepper (if using) to the pot. Stir well to coat the vegetables with the spices.
4. Stir in the cooked lentils, coconut milk, and vegetable broth. Bring the mixture to a boil, then reduce the heat and let it simmer for 25-30 minutes, or until the sweet potatoes are tender.
5. Season the curry with salt and pepper, to taste. Serve the Lentil and Sweet Potato Curry over cooked basmati rice, and enjoy your comforting and nutrient-rich meal!

Mediterranean Chickpea Salad

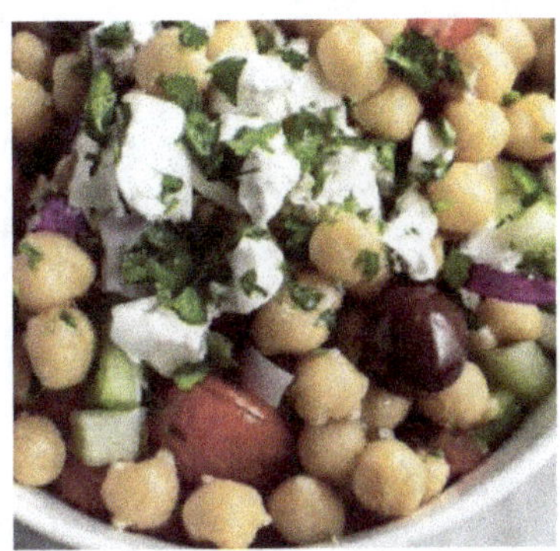

Portion Size: 4 servings

Macronutrient Breakdown (per serving):

- Calories: 350
- Protein: 12g
- Carbohydrates: 40g
- Fat: 17g
- Fibre: 9g

Ingredients:

- 2 (15-ounce) cans chickpeas, rinsed and drained
- 1 cup cherry tomatoes, halved
- 1 large cucumber, diced
- 1/2 red onion, thinly sliced
- 1/2 cup kalamata olives, pitted
- 1/2 cup crumbled feta cheese
- 1/4 cup fresh parsley, chopped

Lemon-Herb Dressing:

- 1/4 cup extra-virgin olive oil
- Juice of 1 lemon
- 1 teaspoon dried oregano
- 1 clove garlic, minced
- Salt and pepper, to taste

Instructions:

1. In a large salad bowl, combine the chickpeas, cherry tomatoes, diced cucumber, thinly sliced red onion, and kalamata olives.

2. In a small bowl or jar, whisk together the extra-virgin olive oil, lemon juice, dried oregano, minced garlic, salt, and pepper to create the lemon-herb dressing.
3. Pour the dressing over the chickpea mixture, and toss well to ensure all the ingredients are coated with the dressing.
4. Top the salad with crumbled feta cheese and chopped fresh parsley. You can serve the Mediterranean Chickpea Salad immediately or refrigerate it for at least an hour to allow the flavours to meld together.
5. Enjoy your delicious and nutritious Mediterranean Chickpea Salad, perfect for a light lunch, side dish, or healthy snack!

Shrimp and Vegetable Stir Fry

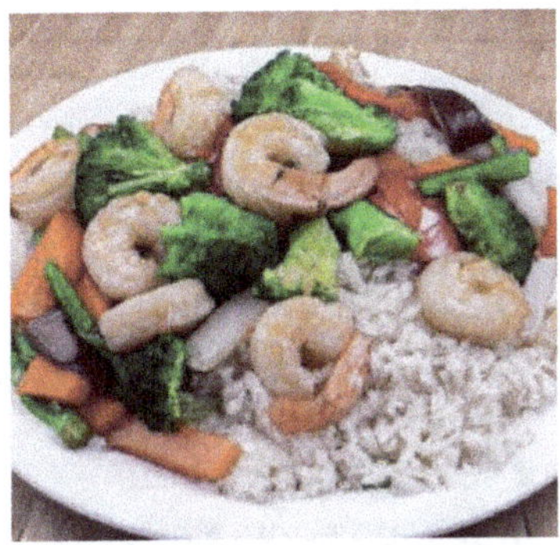

Portion Size: 4 servings

Macronutrient Breakdown (per serving):

- Calories: 350
- Protein: 25g
- Carbohydrates: 40g
- Fat: 9g
- Fibre: 6g

Ingredients:

- 1 pound large shrimp, peeled and deveined
- 2 cups broccoli florets
- 1 cup sliced carrots
- 1 red bell pepper, thinly sliced
- 1 cup snap peas
- 2 tablespoons vegetable oil

Garlic-Ginger Sauce:

- 1/4 cup low-sodium soy sauce
- 2 tablespoons oyster sauce
- 1 tablespoon honey
- 2 cloves garlic, minced
- 1 tablespoon fresh ginger, grated

For serving:

- 4 cups cooked brown rice

Instructions:

1.   In a small bowl, whisk together the low-sodium soy sauce, oyster
      sauce, honey, minced garlic, and grated ginger to create the garlic-
      ginger sauce. Set aside.
2.   In a large skillet or wok, heat 1 tablespoon of vegetable oil over
      medium-high heat. Add the shrimp and cook for 2-3 minutes per side,
      or until pink and cooked through. Transfer the cooked shrimp to a
      plate and set aside.
3.   Add another tablespoon of vegetable oil to the skillet or wok, and add
      the broccoli, carrots, bell pepper, and snap peas. Stir-fry the
      vegetables for 4-5 minutes, or until they are tender-crisp.
4.   Add the cooked shrimp back to the skillet or wok, along with the
      garlic-ginger sauce. Stir well to coat the shrimp and vegetables with
      the sauce, and cook for an additional 1-2 minutes, or until heated
      through.
5.   Serve the Shrimp and Vegetable Stir Fry over cooked brown rice, and
      enjoy your delicious and healthful meal packed with protein and
      vitamins!

Chicken, Avocado, and Strawberry Spinach Salad

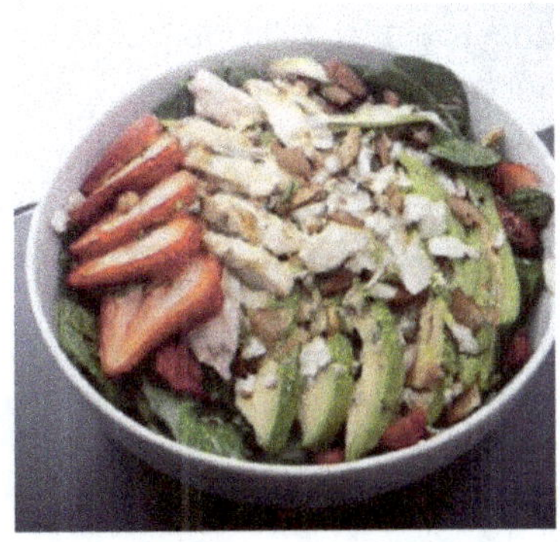

Portion Size: 4 servings

Macronutrient Breakdown (per serving):

- Calories: 385
- Protein: 28g
- Carbohydrates: 18g
- Fat: 25g
- Fibre: 7g

Ingredients:

- 4 cups fresh baby spinach
- 1 pound grilled chicken breast, sliced
- 2 cups fresh strawberries, hulled and halved
- 2 ripe avocados, pitted and sliced
- 1/2 cup crumbled goat cheese
- 1/2 cup toasted almonds

Balsamic Vinaigrette:

- 1/4 cup balsamic vinegar
- 1/2 cup extra-virgin olive oil
- 1 teaspoon Dijon mustard
- 1 tablespoon honey
- Salt and pepper, to taste

Instructions:

1. In a small bowl or jar, whisk together the balsamic vinegar, extra-virgin olive oil, Dijon mustard, honey, salt, and pepper to create the balsamic vinaigrette. Set aside.

2. In a large salad bowl, combine the baby spinach, sliced grilled chicken, halved strawberries, and sliced avocados.

3. Pour the balsamic vinaigrette over the salad, and gently toss to coat all the ingredients with the dressing.

4. Top the salad with crumbled goat cheese and toasted almonds. Serve the Chicken, Avocado, and Strawberry Spinach Salad immediately, and enjoy a refreshing and satisfying meal full of nutrients and flavour!

Zucchini Noodle and Pesto Chicken

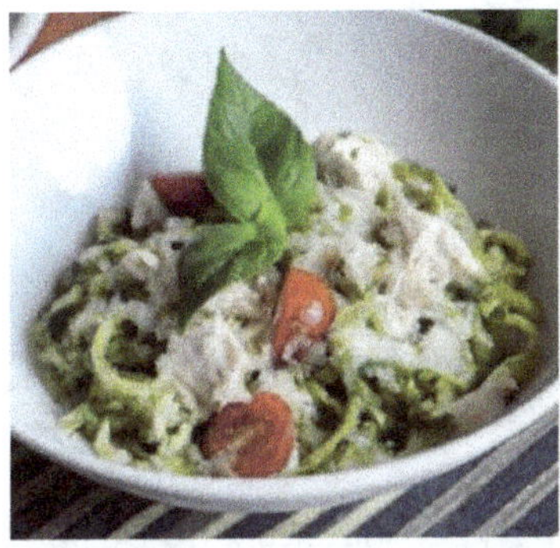

Portion Size: 4 servings

Macronutrient Breakdown (per serving):

- Calories: 410
- Protein: 35g
- Carbohydrates: 14g
- Fat: 24g
- Fibre: 4g

Ingredients:

- 4 medium zucchini, spiralized
- 1 pound boneless, skinless chicken breasts, cubed
- 1 tablespoon olive oil
- Salt and pepper, to taste
- 1 cup cherry tomatoes, halved
- 1/2 cup homemade basil pesto (recipe below)
- Grated Parmesan cheese, for garnish
- Fresh basil leaves, for garnish

Homemade Basil Pesto:

- 2 cups fresh basil leaves
- 1/3 cup pine nuts
- 1/2 cup grated Parmesan cheese
- 2 cloves garlic, minced
- 1/2 cup extra-virgin olive oil
- Salt and pepper, to taste

Instructions:

1. In a food processor, combine the fresh basil leaves, pine nuts, grated Parmesan cheese, and minced garlic. Pulse until coarsely chopped. With the processor running, slowly add the extra-virgin olive oil, and process until smooth. Season the homemade basil pesto with salt and pepper, to taste, and set aside.

2. In a large skillet, heat the olive oil over medium heat. Season the cubed chicken breasts with salt and pepper, and add them to the skillet. Cook the chicken for 6-8 minutes, or until fully cooked and golden brown. Transfer the cooked chicken to a plate and set aside.

3. In the same skillet, add the spiralized zucchini noodles and cook for 3-4 minutes, or until they are just tender. Remove the skillet from the heat and add the cooked chicken, halved cherry tomatoes, and basil pesto. Toss well to combine and coat the zucchini noodles and chicken with the pesto sauce.

4. Serve the Zucchini Noodle and Pesto Chicken in bowls, garnished with grated Parmesan cheese and fresh basil leaves. Enjoy your light and flavourful meal, packed with nutrients and low in carbohydrates!

Spiced Lentil and Sweet Potato Soup

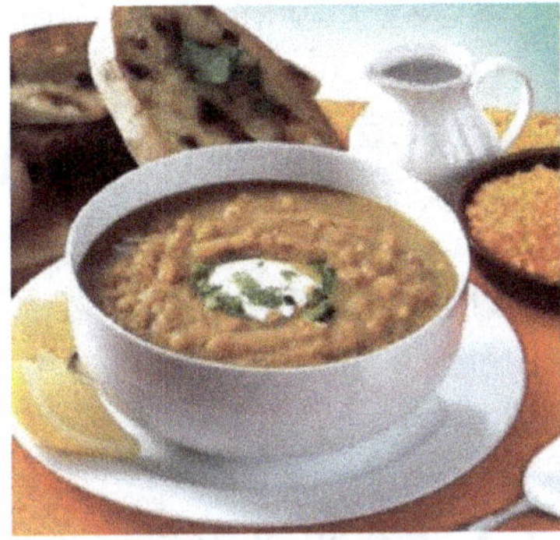

Portion Size: 4 servings

Macronutrient Breakdown (per serving):

- Calories: 365
- Protein: 18g
- Carbohydrates: 60g
- Fat: 6g
- Fibre: 12g

Ingredients:

- 1 tablespoon olive oil
- 1 onion, chopped
- 2 cloves garlic, minced
- 1 tablespoon grated fresh ginger
- 2 teaspoons ground cumin
- 1 teaspoon ground turmeric
- 1/2 teaspoon smoked paprika
- 1 cup red lentils, rinsed and drained
- 1 large sweet potato, peeled and cubed
- 6 cups vegetable broth
- Salt and pepper, to taste

Garnish:

- Chopped fresh cilantro
- Yogurt
- Lemon wedges

For serving:

- Crusty whole-grain bread

Instructions:

1. In a large pot or Dutch oven, heat the olive oil over medium heat. Add the onion and cook for 5-7 minutes, or until softened and translucent.
2. Add the garlic, ginger, cumin, turmeric, and smoked paprika to the pot, and cook for an additional 1-2 minutes, or until fragrant.
3. Stir in the red lentils, cubed sweet potato, and vegetable broth. Bring the mixture to a boil, then reduce the heat to low and simmer for 25-30 minutes, or until the lentils and sweet potatoes are tender.
4. Use an immersion blender to partially blend the soup, leaving some texture. Alternatively, you can carefully transfer about half of the soup to a countertop blender, blend until smooth, and return it to the pot. Season the soup with salt and pepper, to taste.
5. Serve the Spiced Lentil and Sweet Potato Soup hot, garnished with chopped fresh cilantro, a dollop of yogurt, and a lemon wedge. Enjoy your nutritious and comforting meal with crusty whole-grain bread!

Bonus recipes:

Mediterranean Stuffed Bell Peppers

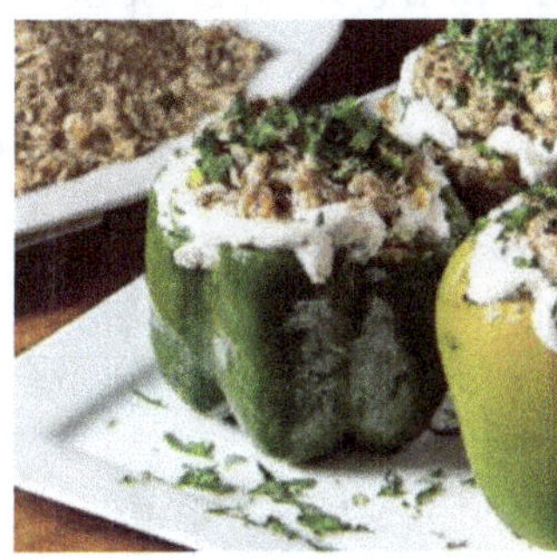

Portion Size: 4 servings

Macronutrient Breakdown (per serving):
- Calories: 410
- Protein: 30g
- Carbohydrates: 34g
- Fat: 18g
- Fibre: 5g

Ingredients:
- 4 large bell peppers (assorted colours), tops removed and seeds cleaned out
- 1 pound ground turkey
- 1 tablespoon olive oil
- 1 onion, diced
- 2 cloves garlic, minced
- 1 cup cooked brown rice
- 2 cups fresh spinach, chopped
- 1 cup crumbled feta cheese
- 1 teaspoon dried oregano
- Salt and pepper, to taste

Garnish:
- Fresh parsley, chopped

For serving:
- Tzatziki sauce

Instructions:

1. Preheat your oven to 375°F (190°C) and prepare a baking dish by lightly greasing it with non-stick spray or oil.
2. In a large skillet, heat the olive oil over medium heat. Add the diced onion and cook for 4-5 minutes, or until softened. Add the garlic and cook for an additional 1 minute, or until fragrant.
3. Add the ground turkey to the skillet, breaking it up with a wooden spoon as it cooks. Cook until the turkey is fully cooked and no longer pink, about 5-7 minutes.
4. Stir in the cooked brown rice, chopped spinach, crumbled feta cheese, dried oregano, salt, and pepper. Cook for an additional 2-3 minutes, or until the spinach is wilted and the mixture is heated through.
5. Stuff the bell peppers with the turkey and rice mixture, filling them to the top. Place the stuffed peppers in the prepared baking dish.
6. Bake the stuffed bell peppers in the preheated oven for 30-35 minutes, or until the bell peppers are tender and the filling is heated through.
7. Remove the Mediterranean Stuffed Bell Peppers from the oven and let them cool for a few minutes before serving. Garnish with chopped fresh parsley and serve with a side of tangy tzatziki sauce. Enjoy your delicious and satisfying high-protein meal!

Baked Lemon Herb Salmon

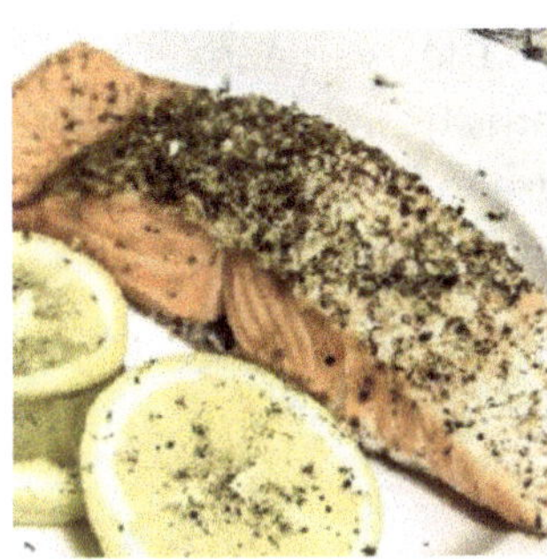

Portion Size: 4 servings

Macronutrient Breakdown (per serving):
- Calories: 435
- Protein: 35g
- Carbohydrates: 30g
- Fat: 21g
- Fibre: 5g

Ingredients:
- 4 (6-ounce) salmon fillets
- Salt and pepper, to taste
- 2 tablespoons olive oil
- 2 cloves garlic, minced
- 1 tablespoon fresh dill, chopped
- 1 tablespoon fresh parsley, chopped
- Zest and juice of 1 lemon
- 1/4 teaspoon crushed red pepper flakes (optional)

For serving:
- Steamed green beans
- Roasted baby potatoes

Instructions:
- 1. Preheat your oven to 400°F (200°C) and line a baking sheet with parchment paper.
- 2. Season the salmon fillets with salt and pepper and place them skin-side down on the prepared baking sheet.
- 3. In a small bowl, mix together the olive oil, minced garlic, chopped dill, chopped parsley, lemon zest, lemon juice, and crushed red pepper flakes (if using).
- 4. Spread the lemon herb mixture evenly over the top of each salmon fillet.

- 5. Bake the salmon fillets in the preheated oven for 12-15 minutes, or until the salmon flakes easily with a fork and reaches an internal temperature of 145°F (63°C).
- 6. Remove the Baked Lemon Herb Salmon from the oven and let it rest for a couple of minutes before serving. Garnish with lemon slices and fresh dill sprigs, and serve with steamed green beans and roasted baby potatoes for a balanced, nutritious meal that's bursting with flavour!

Chicken and Vegetable Stir-Fry

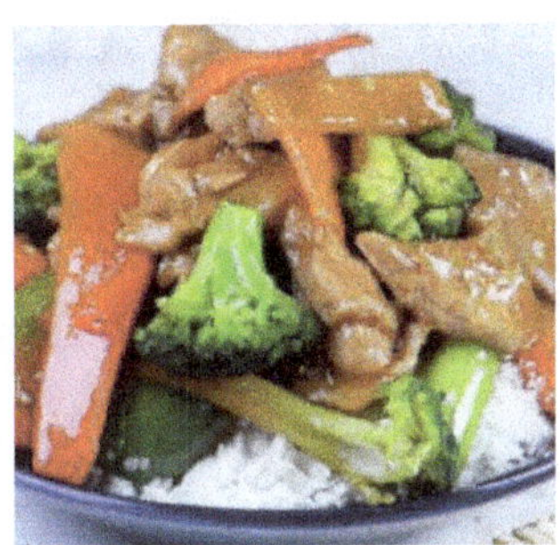

Portion Size: 4 servings

Macronutrient Breakdown (per serving):
- Calories: 430
- Protein: 35g
- Carbohydrates: 47g
- Fat: 12g
- Fibre: 6g

Ingredients:
- 1 pound boneless, skinless chicken breasts, cut into bite-sized pieces
- 2 tablespoons vegetable oil, divided
- 1 red bell pepper, thinly sliced
- 1 yellow bell pepper, thinly sliced
- 2 cups broccoli florets
- 1 cup sliced carrots
- 1/4 cup soy sauce
- 2 tablespoons honey
- 1 tablespoon freshly grated ginger
- 2 cloves garlic, minced
- 1 tablespoon corn starch
- 1/4 cup water

For serving:
- Steamed jasmine rice

Instructions:
1. In a small bowl, whisk together the soy sauce, honey, grated ginger, minced garlic, corn starch, and water until well combined. Set aside.
2. Heat 1 tablespoon of vegetable oil in a large skillet or wok over medium-high heat. Add the chicken pieces and cook until browned and cooked through, about 5-7 minutes. Transfer the cooked chicken to a plate and set aside.

3. In the same skillet, heat the remaining 1 tablespoon of vegetable oil. Add the bell peppers, broccoli, and carrots, and stir-fry for 3-4 minutes, or until the vegetables are crisp-tender.
4. Add the cooked chicken back to the skillet with the vegetables. Pour the soy-ginger sauce over the chicken and vegetables, and cook for an additional 2-3 minutes, or until the sauce has thickened and everything is heated through.
5. Serve the Chicken and Vegetable Stir-Fry over steamed jasmine rice for a satisfying, nutrient-dense meal that's packed with lean protein, vitamins, and minerals!

Turkey Taco Stuffed Zucchini Boats

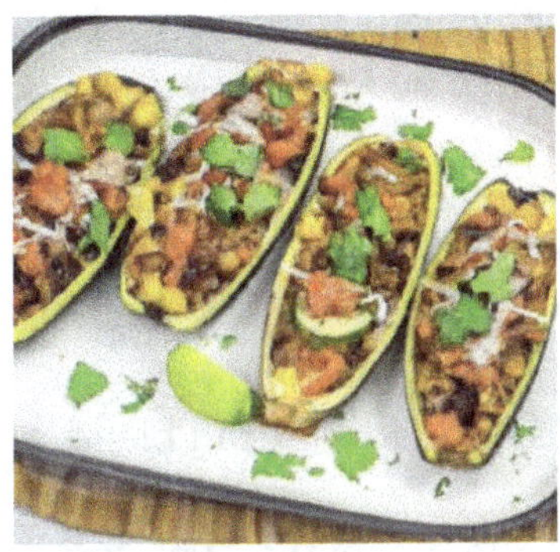

Portion Size: 4 servings (2 zucchini boats per serving)

Macronutrient Breakdown (per serving):
- Calories: 425
- Protein: 36g
- Carbohydrates: 28g
- Fat: 18g
- Fibre: 8g

Ingredients:
- 4 medium zucchini, halved lengthwise
- 1 tablespoon olive oil
- 1 pound ground turkey
- 1 small onion, diced
- 2 cloves garlic, minced
- 1 (15-ounce) can black beans, drained and rinsed
- 1 cup frozen corn, thawed
- 1 (14.5-ounce) can diced tomatoes, drained
- 2 tablespoons taco seasoning
- 1/2 teaspoon salt
- 1 cup shredded Mexican blend cheese

Garnish:
- Fresh cilantro, chopped
- Lime wedges

Instructions:
1. Preheat your oven to 400°F (200°C) and line a large baking sheet with parchment paper or aluminium foil.
2. Using a spoon or melon baller, scoop out the flesh of the zucchini halves, leaving a 1/4-inch thick border. Place the hollowed-out zucchini boats on the prepared baking sheet.

3. In a large skillet, heat the olive oil over medium heat. Add the diced onion and cook for 4-5 minutes, or until softened. Add the garlic and cook for an additional 1 minute, or until fragrant.
4. Add the ground turkey to the skillet, breaking it up with a wooden spoon as it cooks. Cook until the turkey is fully cooked and no longer pink, about 5-7 minutes.
5. Stir in the black beans, corn, diced tomatoes, taco seasoning, and salt. Cook for an additional 2-3 minutes, or until the mixture is heated through.
6. Spoon the turkey taco mixture into the zucchini boats, dividing it evenly among them. Top each zucchini boat with shredded Mexican blend cheese.
7. Bake the Turkey Taco Stuffed Zucchini Boats in the preheated oven for 20-25 minutes, or until the zucchini is tender and the cheese is melted and bubbly.
8. Remove the zucchini boats from the oven and let them cool for a few minutes before serving. Garnish with chopped fresh cilantro and serve with lime wedges for a fresh, nutritious, and high-protein meal!

Mediterranean Chicken and Couscous Salad

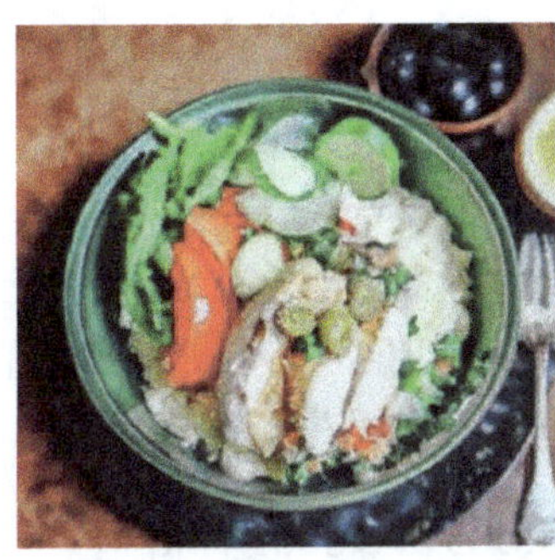

Portion Size: 4 servings

Macronutrient Breakdown (per serving):
- Calories: 435
- Protein: 32g
- Carbohydrates: 50g
- Fat: 14g
- Fibre: 5g

Ingredients:
- 1 pound boneless, skinless chicken breasts
- Salt and pepper, to taste
- 1 cup uncooked couscous
- 1 cup cherry tomatoes, halved
- 1 cup diced cucumber
- 1/2 cup pitted Kalamata olives, halved
- 1/2 cup crumbled feta cheese
- 1/4 cup chopped fresh parsley

Lemon-Tahini Dressing:
- 3 tablespoons tahini
- 3 tablespoons lemon juice
- 1 tablespoon olive oil
- 2 cloves garlic, minced
- Salt and pepper, to taste

Instructions:

1. Preheat your grill or grill pan to medium-high heat. Season the chicken breasts with salt and pepper and cook them for 5-7 minutes per side, or until they are fully cooked and have an internal temperature of 165°F (74°C). Let the chicken rest for a few minutes before slicing into bite-sized pieces.

2. Cook the couscous according to the package instructions. Fluff it with a fork and let it cool slightly.
3. In a small bowl, whisk together the tahini, lemon juice, olive oil, minced garlic, salt, and pepper until smooth. Set the Lemon-Tahini Dressing aside.
4. In a large bowl, combine the cooked couscous, sliced grilled chicken, cherry tomatoes, diced cucumber, Kalamata olives, and crumbled feta cheese. Drizzle the Lemon-Tahini Dressing over the salad and toss gently to combine.
5. Divide the Mediterranean Chicken and Couscous Salad among four bowls and garnish with chopped fresh parsley. Enjoy this protein-rich, flavour-packed salad that's perfect for a nutritious and satisfying fitness meal!